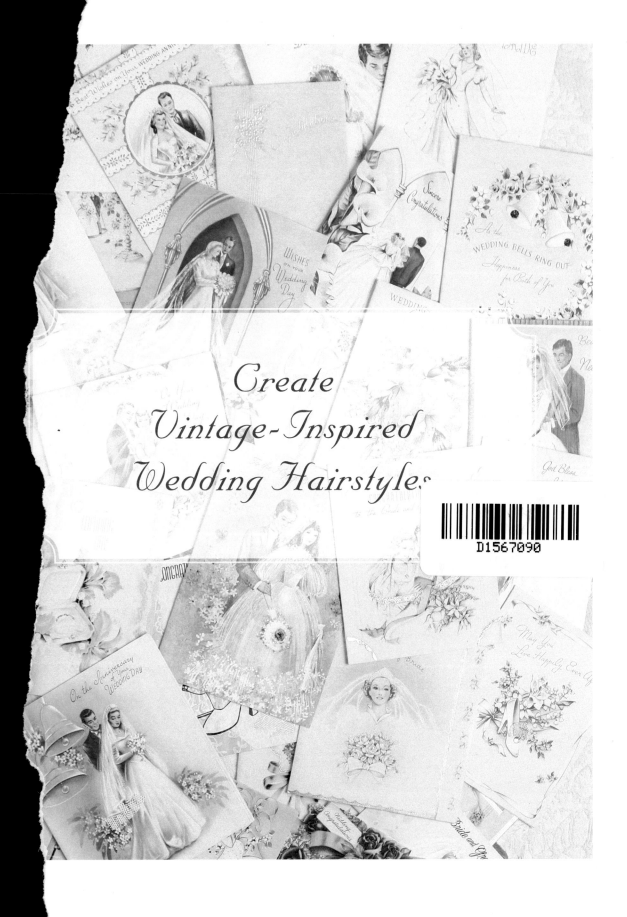

Create
Vintage-Inspired
Wedding Hairstyles

D1567090

Dedication

For my grandparents, Mae, Keith, J. A., and Marian.

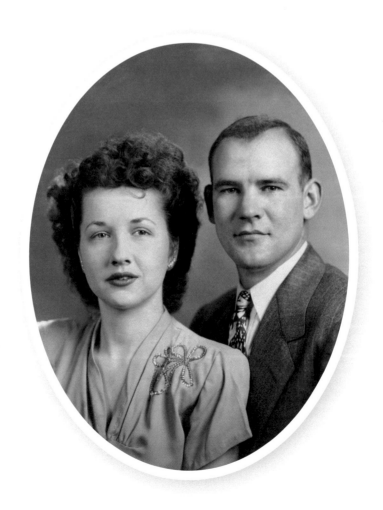

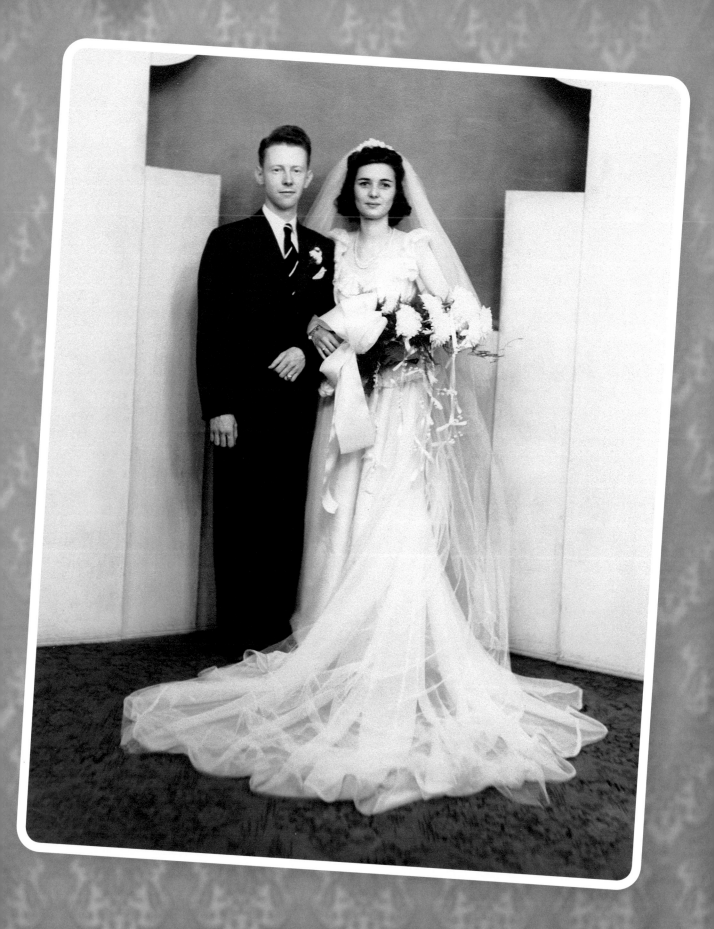

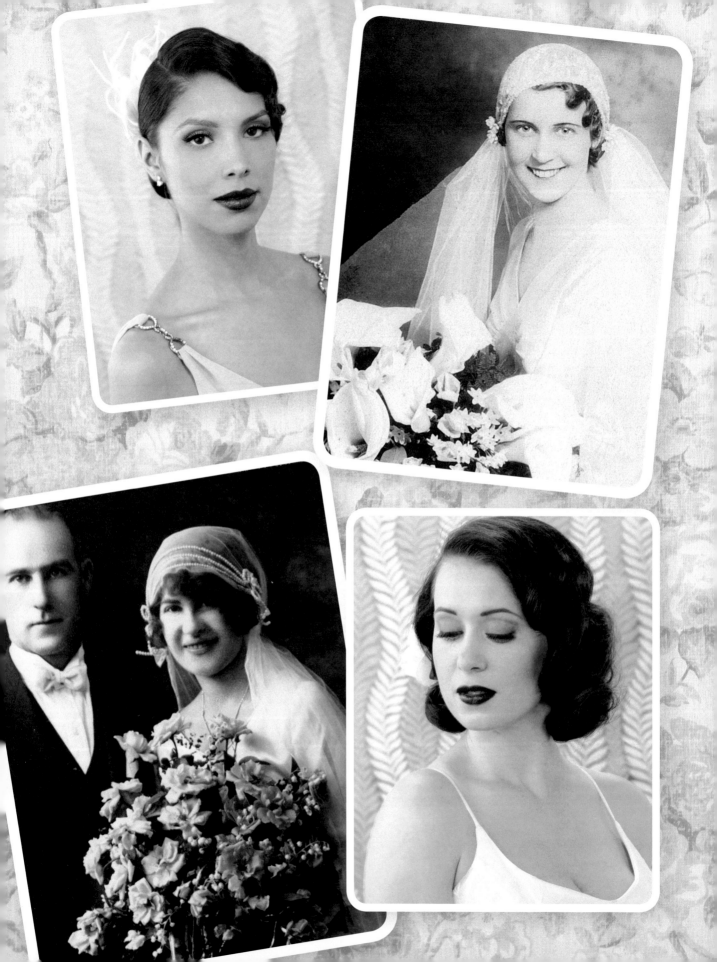

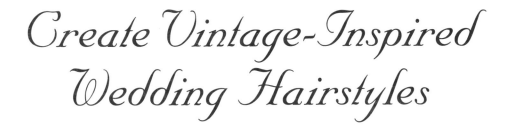

Create Vintage-Inspired Wedding Hairstyles

A Step-by-Step Guide to Styling Classic Hairstyles for Any Special Occasion
including Weddings, Proms, and Formal Events

By Lauren Rennells

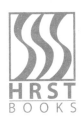

HRST
BOOKS

Cover Design by Benjamin Rennells
Photography © 2014 by Lauren Rennells unless noted in image credits

Published by HRST Books
Post Office Box 18429
Denver, Colorado 80218-8429 U.S.A.
info@hrstbooks.com; www.hrstbooks.com

Library of Congress Cataloging-in-Publication Data
Rennells, Lauren.
  Create Vintage-Inspired Wedding Hairstyles: A Step-by-Step Guide to Styling Classic Hairstyles for Any Special Occasion including Weddings, Proms, and Formal Events / by Lauren Rennells
220 p. 26 cm.
ISBN-13: 978-0-9816639-3-7
1. Hairdressing. 2. Hairstyles. 3. Weddings I. Title.

Library of Congress Control Number: 2014918999

Printed in the United States of America

Notice to Readers

The reader is encouraged to take all safety precautions in performing any techniques or activities herein. By following the instructions the reader or anyone acting on behalf of the reader willingly assumes all risks of harm in connection with performing these techniques. The author and HRST Books are not liable or responsible to any person or entity with respect to any loss or damage caused, or alleged to have been caused, directly or indirectly, by the information contained in this book.

Acknowledgments

I am grateful for everyone who helped make this book possible. First on the list is Rich for being my best friend and for also being so patient with me and my absence while writing. Thank you to Yara for working so hard and keeping this enterprise afloat. Thank you to my parents for guiding me and standing with me on my journey. Thank you to my brothers and sister for so much and my friends for being my cheerleaders through this process.

A special thanks to my many mentors along my path including Miss Lil and Miss Cindy, Dena Olivett, Sharon Blain, Paula Hibbard, Davida Simon, Leslie Snyder, Jenece Amella, Lorraine Altamura and the many other beauty professionals I have had the honor of learning from, working along side of, and have been inspired by.

Thank you to all of the very beautiful models that sat for the book including Kira, Lindsay, Nieve, Laura, Victoria, Katy, Rebecca, and Keira, and the women of history in images scattered throughout the book. Your lovely faces make this book as beautiful as it can be.

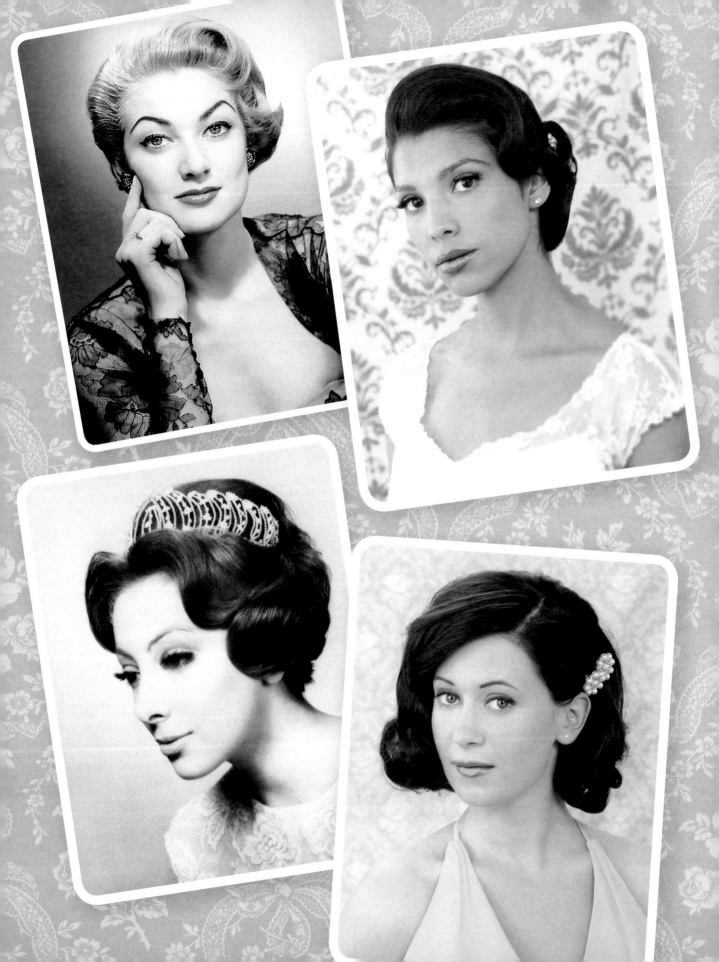

Contents

Hairstyle Steps

Introduction

You have made most of the major decisions about your special day: the colors, the dress, the flowers. Now it is time to plan for a key element to your perfect day: your hair. You have spent the last 6 months trying to grow it as long as possible and have set the appointment with the hairstylist for a color retouch. But you still have some planning to do, because you have decided you want a vintage hairstyle on your wedding day. Whether your entire wedding is based around the art deco 1930s, you are having a rockabilly wedding at an amusement park, or you consider your wedding modern, but love the glamour of days-gone-by.

Now where do you start? What do you mean by vintage? You are wearing your grandmother's 1940s biased cut gown, but she wore her hair up and you want to wear yours down. You saw a picture online you really liked, but you are not sure how to get a curl like it. You have this vision in your head, but you have no idea how to begin.

In *Create Vintage-Inspired Wedding Hairstyles*, my attempt is to bring together my love of classic beauty, my obsession with designing hairstyles, and my years of striving to make brides happy and beautiful. My hope in the end is that you find the hairstyle of your dreams in these pages or the skills you need to create what you have been envisioning in your head to be the perfect hairstyle.

The book is filled with step-by-step instructions for beautiful, formal hairstyles inspired by the forms and silhouettes worn by women from the Victorian and Edwardian eras, the 1920s, 30s, 40s, 50s, and 60s. The styles are not designed to be exact replicas of hairstyles from these time periods, but to be fresh, modern revivals of the glamour and romance. I share the who's, what's, where's, why's, and how's that led to the final designs that will hopefully help you take your inspiration piece and interpret it into exactly what you dreamed in your own mind.

Your memories of your wedding day will make it seem as if it were just yesterday. You will also have the photographs to look through for years to come and vintage touches like your hairstyle will make your wedding appear timeless… just like it is in your own memory.

Lauren Rennells

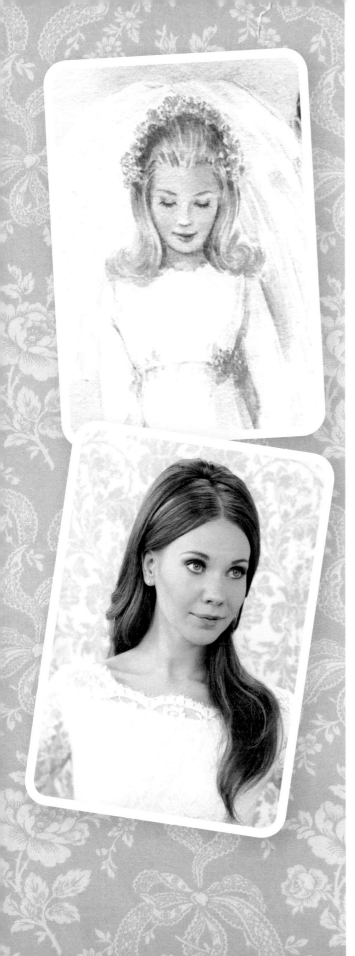

What is *Vintage* vs. *Vintage-Inspired?*

Before we begin, let's clarify the difference between "vintage" and "vintage-inspired" as it pertains to this book. Not because there is a right way or a wrong way, but because it will greatly help narrow in on what the final style should look like and in communication between hairstylist and hair client.

The word "vintage" can be a serious subject. To some the word is very sacred. It is used to describe items or techniques truly from the time period. To other people, vintage can mean something that was replicated to look like the time period. To others still, vintage is a loose term that refers to the romantic, delicate appearance of time-gone-by and they do not necessarily equate it with any particular point in time.

It is important to define what the word means to you, your client, your hairstylist, or anyone else that is involved in the process of the final hairstyle. Everyone should be on the same page to get an end result everyone is happy with.

When I use the word "vintage" as it pertains to hairdressing, it generally means to me more of a replication type scenario. "Vintage-inspired" is truly just that...inspired by the past. The hairstyles of this book use profiles, silhouettes, and textures to nod back to various decades of the late 19th thru mid-20th Centuries without attempting full replicas. I find these types of hairstyles work wonderful for the majority of brides I work with who are looking for a "vintage" hairstyle for their wedding day.

Choosing
your inspiration

You know you want "vintage", but how do you decide what the hairstyle should look like? The first step is getting a feel for what you like. You may already have done this. You have a picture of your grandmother with her soldier husband or a picture of your favorite movie star from the 1950s. You may even have a whole crop of images you pinned when you put in a search for finger wave hairstyles. Inspiration for a uniquely-you hairstyle can come from anywhere.

The internet is a great place to start in your search, but in a quest for that unique day you have always dreamed of, I encourage you to step outside of the currently-popular box. Go through your family photo albums, your grandfather's college yearbook, or the local antique store's selection of vintage photographs. You may see an element of something you had not considered.

This book is certainly designed to provide you with the experience of picking a style, pointing to it, and saying, "I want my hair to look like this." This book is also designed to help you get between points *A* and *B*: *A* being a vintage image of a vintage hairstyle that makes you happy and *B* being a flattering, long-lasting hairstyle that captures the classic beauty you are striving for.

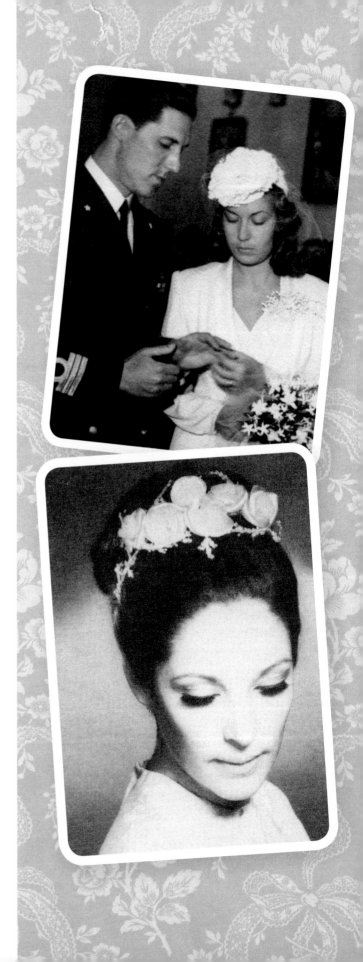

Considering your inspiration

What do you see in your inspiration? What is drawing your eye to it? What is it in this style that you would like to recreate or emulate?

   Start with simple answers. It is a hairstyle from the decade the wedding has been fashioned after. The wave is pretty. It will allow me to wear the decorative hair pick I have already bought.

   As you answer these questions, the foundation for what you want will start to shape up and give you a better vocabulary to define what your final hairstyle should look like.

   As always, be realistic when you see something you really like. Ask yourself if it is truly possible based on what the hair you are working with can do and remember a lot can be accomplished if you are open to adjustments. You will see in the following pages, with a little creativity, much is possible. Long hair can be made to look short. Fine hair can be made to look thick. Shorter hair can be styled into an up-do.

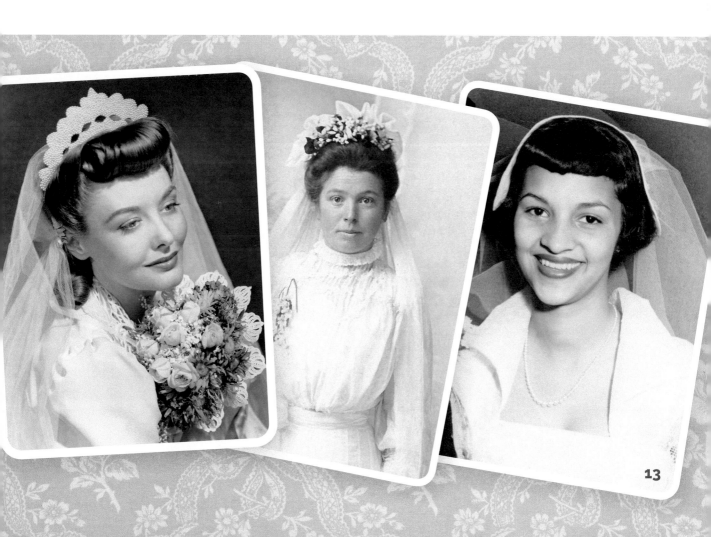

Designing from your inspiration

There are 5 important elements to consider in the design of a great formal hairstyle, especially a vintage-inspired one: the silhouette, interior, texture, movement, and focal point.

- The **form** or **silhouette** of a hairstyle refers to the visible shape of the style. Imagine looking at the hairstyle from a few different directions and drawing a line around the outside of it. Where would that line curve out away from the scalp or neck? Where would that line follow the form of the head? How high would that line be above the forehead?

- The **interior** is the inside of the hairstyle that makes up everything that is happening inside the silhouette.

- **Texture** is defined as "the feel, appearance, or consistency of a surface or a substance." When the word is used in relation to hairstyles it can refer to different things. The texture of a person's hair can be fine, medium, or coarse. Texture can refer to how the state of the cuticle of the hair shaft makes the hair feel to the touch. If the cuticle is closed, the hair feels smooth. If the cuticle is open or damaged it feels a little rougher. Texture also relates to the level of curl or lack there of in a hairstyle.

- The **movement** or **direction** describes where the hairstyle is going. What direction is the hairstyle taking your eyes? Are your eyes being drawn to the back of the style? Are your eyes being drawn to the eyes of the wearer? Movement and direction add texture to a hairstyle as well in things like waves and rolls.

- A **focal point** is defined as "the center or point of interest." In a hairstyle, a focal point can be obvious or subtle, but it should have one. Look through the styles in this book and see if you can determine their focal points. Some are more impactful than others, but each one has elements that draw your eye to them. When you are choosing a vintage hairstyle for your inspiration, look for styles that have a focal point that draws in your own eye.

On the opposite page, see the inspiration piece for the Elizabeth hairstyle. It is a drawing from an 1864 issue of *The Queen, The Ladies' Newspaper and Court Chronicle*.
Since this is a drawing from a very old newspaper, there is a lot left open to interpretation. You will find this often in inspiration images. A bride in a photograph from 1928 may be wearing a very full veil or a photograph from 1942 could be blurry, but that is where the creativity and the fun come in.
Every hairstyle is open to many options. Be creative with the possibilities.

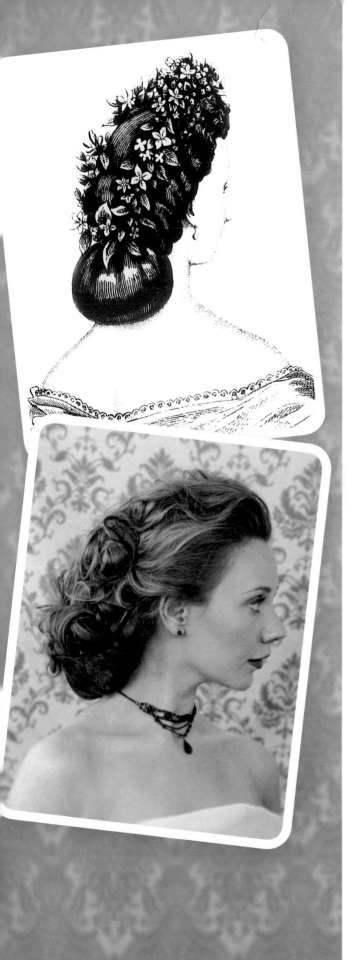

From this...

The first thing in this Victorian hairstyle to consider is the **silhouette**, since it is the dominating element of the drawing. It is focused on the lower back of the head. It does not come over the face and it is round at the base of the neck.

Next consider the **focal point**. The drawing actually has a couple. All the **texture** created by the flowers is a focal point, along with the large bun shape.

Last consider the **movement**. The flowers of the hairstyle not only create the texture, but also the movement as they cascade down the back of it.

This drawing is not descriptive enough to give us the **interior**, so the interior will be determined as an effect of bringing all of the other elements into the hairstyle.

...To this

These elements are all interpretted into the final style to the left.

In the original image it looks like some volume and texture that sits on the head is focused more around the perimeter by the face. I changed that up and opted to keep the sides a little smoother and sweep them back. Sweeping back hair draws the eyes back which adds a face lift effect and enhances the cheekbones.

Instead of covering the back of the head with flowers, the loose, unkempt curl adds the same cascading texture.

For the focal point of the large bun shape at the nape of the neck, I enlarged it even more. A bride is photographed from all angles and by enlarging the bun, it can also be seen a little from the front.

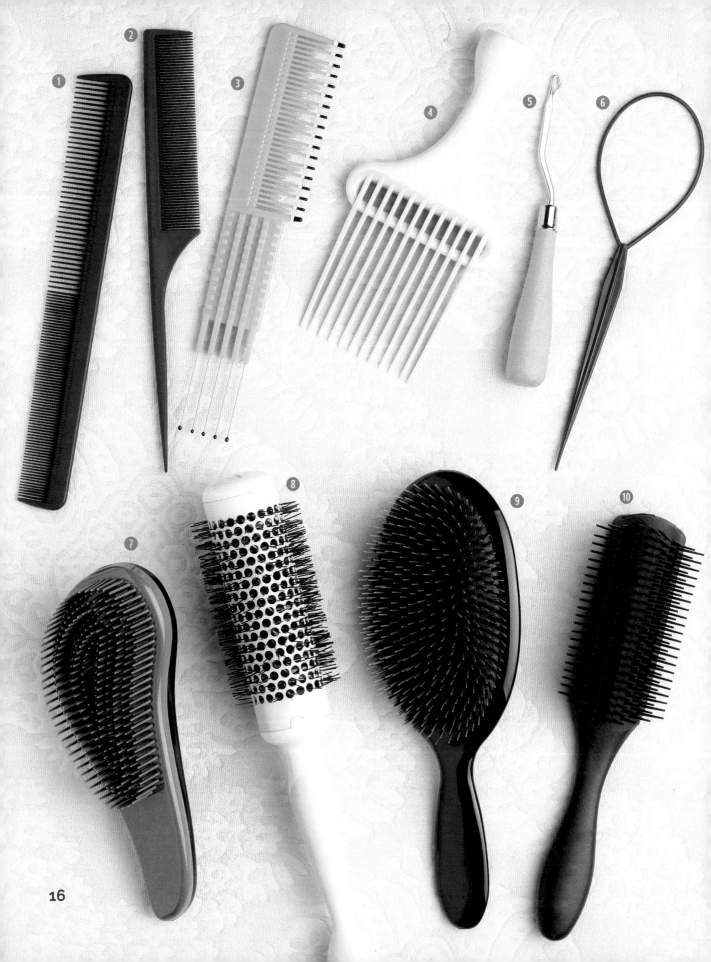

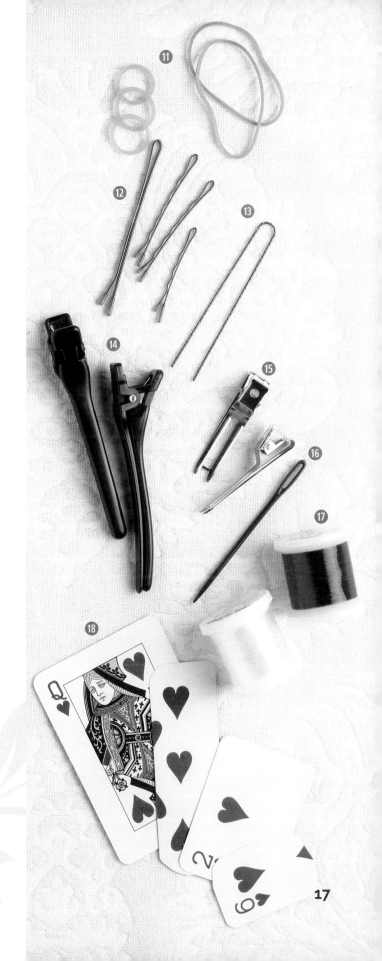

1 **Carbon cutting comb** - Carbon resists heat and grips better than plastic

2 **Carbon tail comb** - Use to separate hair into sections

3 **Wide tooth teasing comb** - For teasing, combing, and lifting

4 **Hair pik** - For combing curls gently

5 **Latch hook tool** - Available from the craft store

6 **Loop and tail styling tool** - Better known as topsy tail, available online

7 **Detangle teaser brush** - Has plastic teeth that bend easily

8 **Round vent brush** - For blow dry styling

9 **Natural bristle grooming brush** - Available from most beauty supply

10 **Styling brush** - Bristles are harder and do not bend

11 **Elastic bands** - Small braid bands and larger #16 bands from the office store

12 **Grib bob pins** - Small, medium, and large

13 **Ripple hair pins** - The wire of the pins is textured for grip

14 **Duckbill clips** - Plastic or metal

15 **Hair clips** - Hold small amounts of hair while styling

16 **2 ¾" plastic craft needle** - Available in craft stores

17 **Lightweight monofilament line** - Available at the craft store

18 **Playing cards** - Cut into thin strips, help form waves and protect hair

17

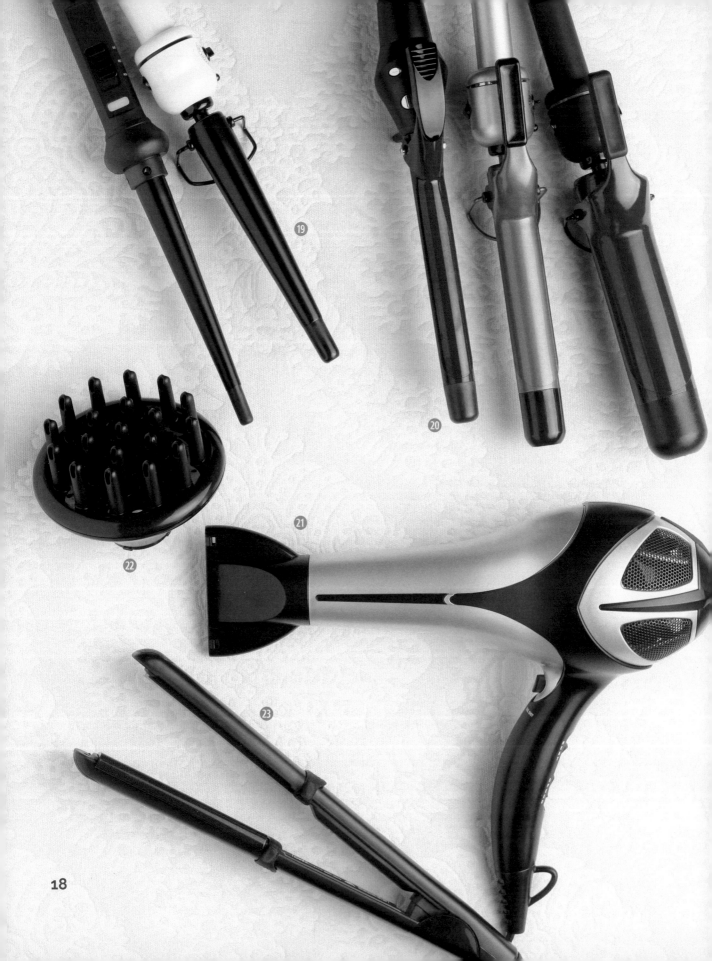

19

20

21

22

23

18

19 **Tapered curling irons** - Come in various widths, suggest finger protection

20 **Curling irons** - Spring or marcel style

21 **Hair dryer with nozzle** - Should have multiple heat settings

22 **Diffuser attachment** - Aids styling by adding heat to curls and waves

23 **Straightening iron** - Should have temperature control to protect hair

24 **Hot rollers** - Set should have small, medium, and large rollers

25 **Hot sticks** - Special bending hot curlers

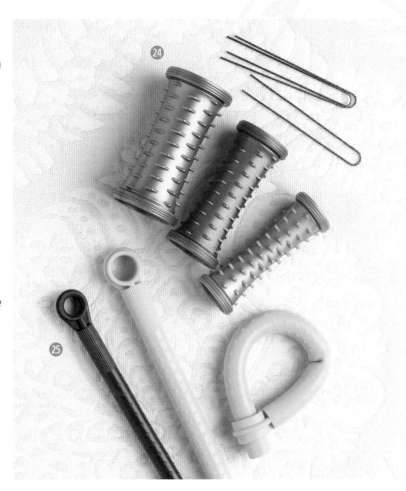

Tips

26 Ripple pins are helpful to keep hot rollers from unraveling.

27 Insert the ripple pin in different directions into the hair wrapped around the hot roller. The placement of the hot roller can determine a different angle for hold.

28 For better curl with rollers, use hot heat from hair dryer with diffuser attachment direct on hair around rollers. Then allow hair to cool before removing rollers.

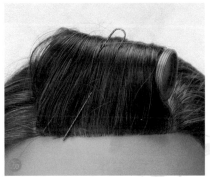

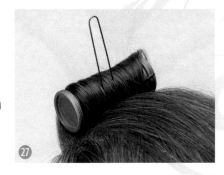

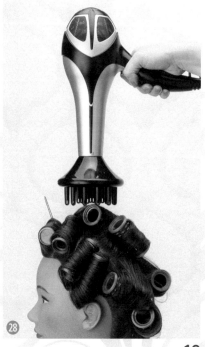

Tapered Curling Iron

The tapered curling iron is used for a few styles in this book. The curl created with this tool has more of a wave effect than a traditional curling iron.

It differs from a traditional curling iron because the wand tapers down in width from base to tip. The most common sizes are ¾ tapered to ½ inch, 1 tapered to ½ inch, and 1¼ tapered to ¾ inch. It is important to choose the right wand size for the desired style. Each style in this book specifies the wand size for the best results.

The tapered wand does not have a shell like a curling iron and so the hair must be wrapped by hand. Until comfortable with the use of this tool, it is highly recommended you use the heat resistant glove that comes with the tool to protect your fingers.

There are 2 directions to wrap the hair around the wand depending on the side of the head you are working on and the desired effect. The first explained here is the right wrap pattern. I often use this pattern when I am working on the left side of the head. The left wrap pattern I use more often on the right side of the head. In my experience, this placement creates a prettier effect around the hairline at the face.

Right Wrap Pattern

1 Begin with a square section of hair in your right hand that is the size of the larger end of the wand. The curling iron held by your left hand is held close to the scalp with out touching it. Begin wrapping the hair at the larger base end of the wand.

2 Wrap the hair section over the top of the wand and under to the right.

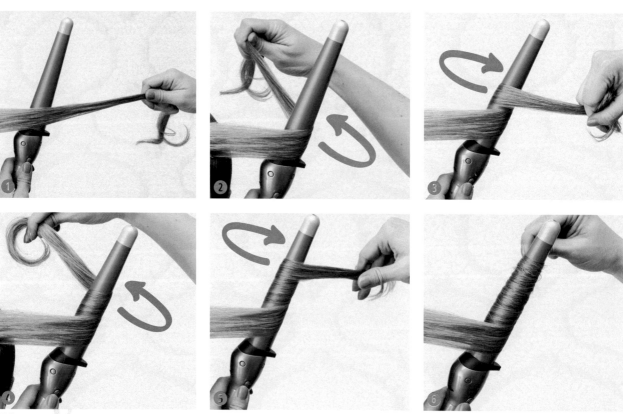

3 Wrap the hair section back over the wand and to the right. With each wrap around the curling iron, the hair moves to the right along the wand and does not overlap the previous wrap around.

4 Also, be sure not to twist the hair section while you are wrapping. Imagine it is a ribbon that you are trying to wrap flat around the wand.

5 Continue to wrap the hair around and down the tapered wand.

6 When you reach the end of the section, keep the ends of the hair between your fingers. Once heated throughly, remove the curl and pin in place with a hair clip to cool. Use caution not to burn your fingers.

Left Wrap Pattern

7 The left wrap pattern follows the same steps as the right except you will hold the curling iron in your right hand and use your left hand to wrap the hair section around the wand and to the left.

8 Wrap the hair section over the top of the wand and under to the left.

9 Wrap the hair section back over the wand and to the left.

10-12 Continue the same as steps 4-6 of the right hair wrap pattern, but wrapping left down the wand. Pin in place with a hair clip to cool. Use caution not to burn your fingers.

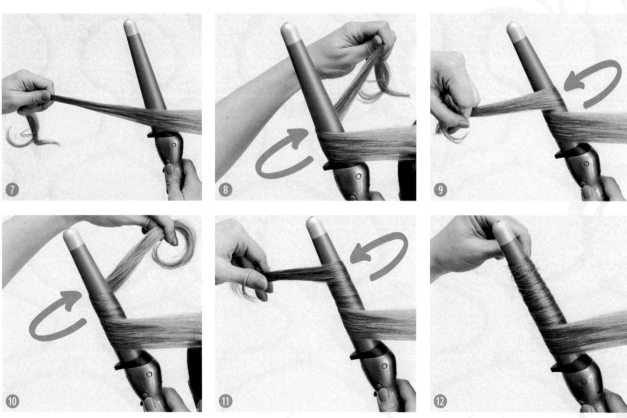

Hair Prep and Pre-Style Treatment

There are many important things to consider for a bridal or event hairstyle. For one, the treatment of the hair before you start the style has a huge effect on the finished appearance.

This pre-treament can include how the hair was treated all day before you even sat down to do the hair. If you let hair air dry flat against the scalp, you will fight to get the volume you may want. There could be a strange hairgrowth pattern that works against you or you may need to move the part for a different effect.

This is where prepping the hair properly for styling will save you, your frustration, and the finished hairstyle.

1 For volume and life in the hairstyle, prep the base of the scalp with volumizing product.

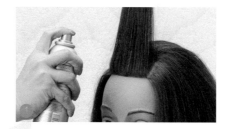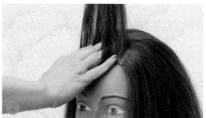

2 Massage the product in and gently tug the hair outward away from the scalp.

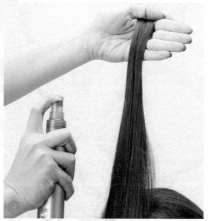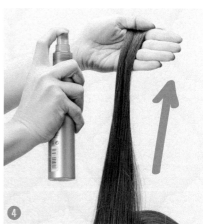

3 Next add thermal styling product to the midshaft and ends of the hair.

4 In sections, spray thermal setting spray from root to tip. For a special event, I like to use 4-5 sprays of product to get a good coat over the hair. It adds stamina and makes it easier control to the hair.

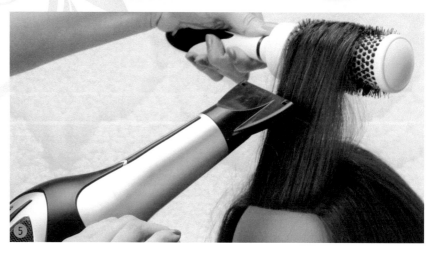

5 Using a vented round brush, set the sprays you just used into the hairshaft. Spray more thermal spray at the start of the curl process.

Base Direction Blow-Dry

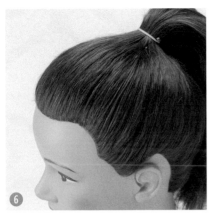

It is important that the hair at the base of the scalp flows in the right direction for a hairstyle. In this example, image number 6 shows a ponytail without proper base direction. There are lumps and the strands are competing with each other to lay flat.

7,8 To remedy this, spray the base of a section of hair with thermal styling spray. Pressing the hair flat with a carbon comb, blow dry small sections in the direction the style will set.

9 The hair will lay cleaner.

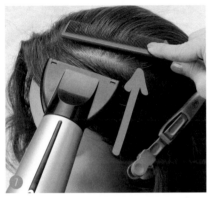

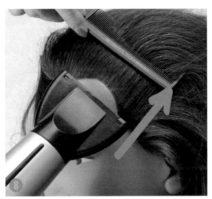

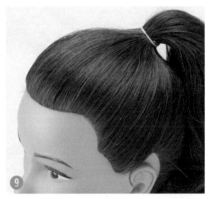

The same principal can be used to define a part or make a part disappear.

10 Spray the base of a section of hair with thermal styling spray.

11 Pressing the hair with a carbon comb, blow dry the hair around the part flat to define the part.

12 To camouflage a part, spray the base of the part with thermal styling spray.

13 Massage the product in and gently tug the hair outward while blow-drying.

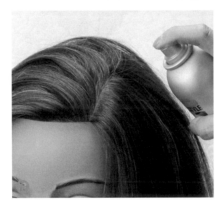

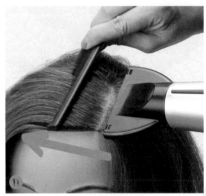

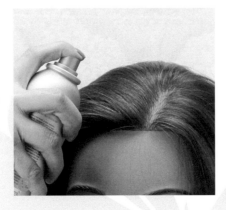

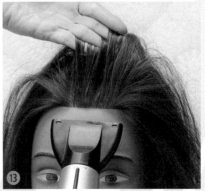

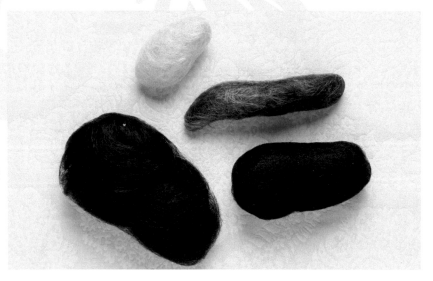

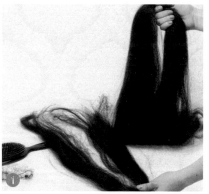

Hair Filler

Often known as hair rats, hair fillers are unbelievably useful for formal vintage hairstyles. They create the illusion of more hair. They provide volume and control. They also provide extra grip for bob pins to hold on to.

I have a small assortment I have ready made. I prefer to make my own when I can. It allows me to make any shape or size I want and I can cater the color to the hair. In general it is better for the hair filler to be 1 or 2 shades darker than the haircolor of the hair it is going to be styled into.

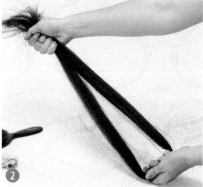

The supplies you will need are:
1. **inexpensive braiding material** found at most consumer beauty supply shops by the extensions
2. **natural bristle grooming brush**
3. **hair net with elastic**

1 Separate a section of braiding hair out of the package.

2 Double it over into a loop.

3 Vigorously back-brush the hair.

4 Continue to back-brush knotting it into a bulky mass.

5 Fold the mass over to condense its shape.

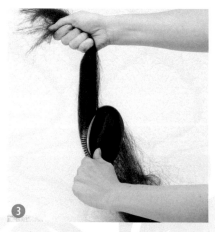

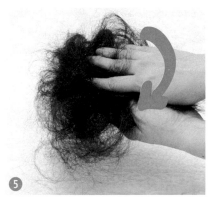

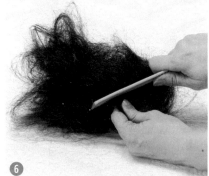

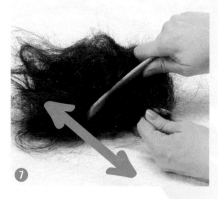

6,7 Use a teasing comb to tease, refine the shape, and create density in the mass.

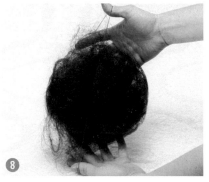

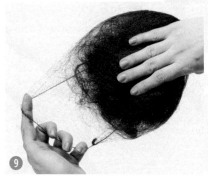

8 Wrap a hair net with elastic around the mass.

9 Use you fingers to tuck the hair into the net.

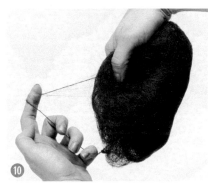

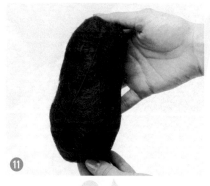

10,11 Continue to pull an edge of the hair net around the mass pressing with your fingers to refine the shape.

Alternative Tip

It is possible to use your own hair for a filling if you are in a pinch and do not have the braiding material on hand.

12 Back-brush a hair section.

13 Wrap a hair net around it.

14 Pin the form into position.

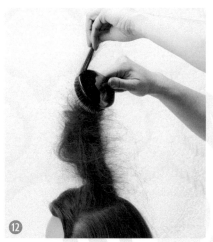

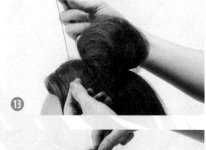

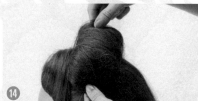

25

Sewing Hair

The purpose of sewing the hair is to provide more hold without the need for tremendous amounts of bob pins. It is also a great tool for manipulating the form of a hairstyle as is used in the Celia and the Victoria hairstyles ahead in the book.

In the steps below, regular thread is being used for visual purposes. Monofilament is best to use because it disappears into the hair, which is exactly what you want.

1. Only use a ¾" plastic craft needle for this for safety. With a 3 foot long piece of monofilament, thread the plastic needle and double over the thread. Tie the 2 ends together in a double knot.

2. Insert the needle near the scalp where it will be hidden in the finished hairstyle. Then insert the needle between the two sides of the knotted monofilament ends.

3. Pull craft needle through and tighten. This is the beginning of the sew line.

4. Begin to "sew" the craft needle through the section of hair you want to hold in place. This is a great way to help hold a wave in place.

5. Sewing can also be used to hold dry pin curls in place without unsightly bob pins.

6. Stop when you have about 3 inches of monofilament at the end. You will need it to tie off the end so the sewing does not unravel.

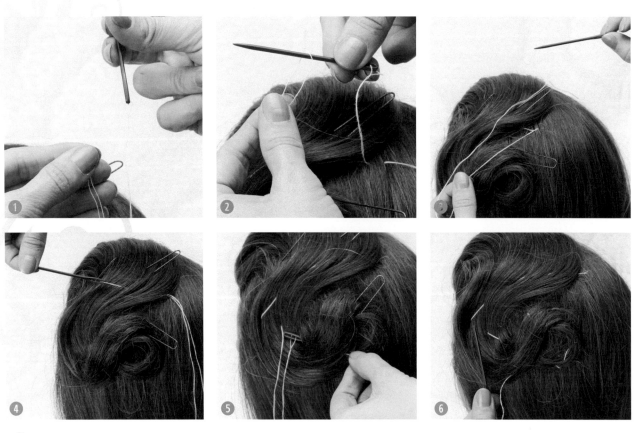

Ponytail

There are a few hairstyles ahead in the book that use ponytails. When securing larger sections of hair into a ponytail, it is easy for hair to slip out of place. With the proceeding method, your ponytail will stay as lovely as it was when you brushed it into your hands.

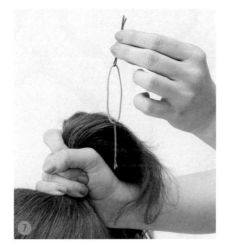

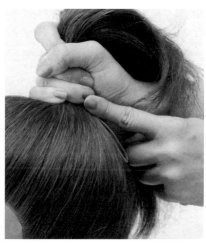

7 Start with a #16 size rubberband from the office supply and 2 grip bob pins attached to the band.

8 Keeping your hand tight around the ponytail, insert one of the bob pins into the base of the ponytail.

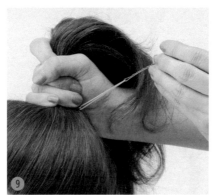

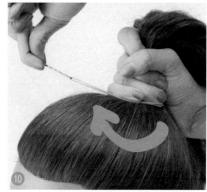

9 Grab the other bob pin.

10 Using the bob pin, pull the rubberband around the base of the ponytail under your hand.

11 Continue the rotation.

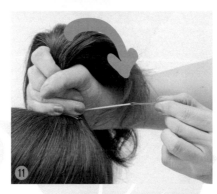

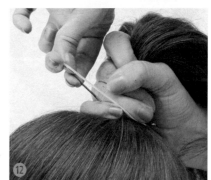

12 Pull the rubberband over to the other side from where the first bob pin was placed. You now should have made 1 ½ rotations around.

13 Insert the second bob pin into the base.

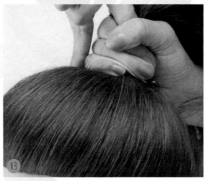

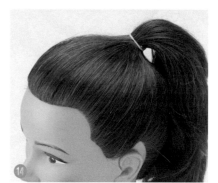

Other Tips and Tidbits

There are many tricks you can use to make your hairstyles better and your life easier. I encourage you to read through this entire book and all the steps of the various hairstyles. Even if it is not the hairstyle you are trying to accomplish, you never know if there is a tidbit in it that will make your current project easier to acheive.

1 A great way to give extra setting power to a hairstyle when it is finished is to use hot heat from a hair dryer with the diffuser attachment. After you have created a wave and clipped it in place for setting like the Hazel or Rose hairstyles further ahead in the book, heat the wave up. Then allow hair to cool before removing the cards and clips.

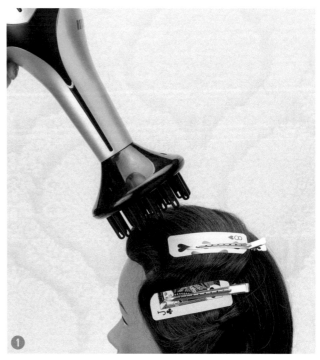

2 Ripple pins are very helpful in holding a style in place or manipulating a section while you are working.

3 While you are styling a section, if you want the hair to stay, but you are not quite ready to grip pin it in place, use the ripple pin as a temporary secure. When you are ready to pin or sew for permanent hold, just place the grip bob pins where the ripple pins are and then remove the ripple pins.

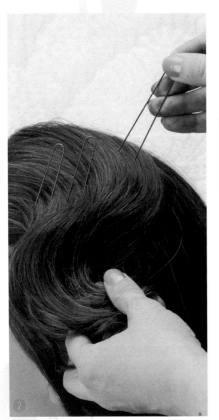
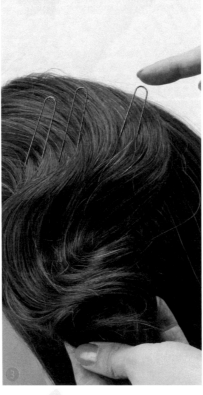

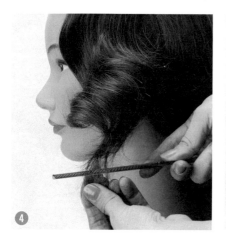 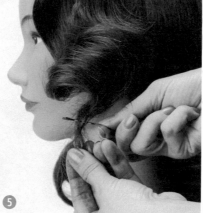 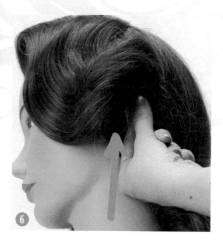

4 Some hair ends that need to be grip pinned into the hairstyle have a tendency to slip out of their pin. To remedy this, use a comb to tease the ends and lock them to each other.

5 Then reinsert the grip bob pin through the teased ends.

6 Pin the piece hidden away in the hairstyle.

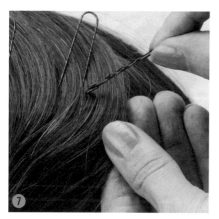 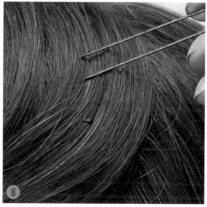 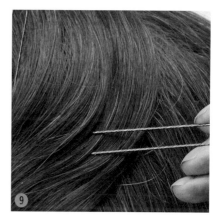

7 After you have gotten the style in position insert the grip bob pins for long term hold.

8 Remove the ripple pin you were using to hold your manipulations.

9 Use the ends of the ripple pin to manipulate a small amount of hair over to cover the grip pin you just secured with. Lightly spray with lightweight hairspray.

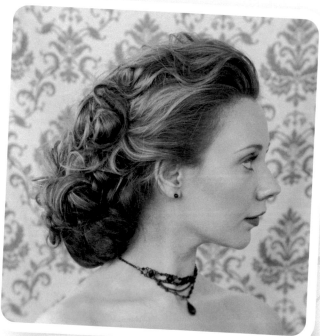

Elizabeth is a modern interpretation of a Victorian era hairstyle. It is the earliest inspired in the book and combines a few facets of the Victorian ideal of beautiful hair.

Victorian women were known for growing their hair as long as possible. Long, healthy hair was a sign of good health and wealth. They curled their valuable hair in rollers made from ripped up pieces of cloth, called rag rollers, and then pinned these beautiful curls up into elaborate hairstyles.

Hair was actually worth money. Hair pieces were sold to add fullness to these elaborate hairstyles and wealthy women would spend a lot on quality pieces. In the book Little Women, by Louisa May Alcott, first published in 1868, the character Jo actually sells her hair to help her family with money troubles.

This hairstyle is meant to be full with lots of wavy texture. To add to the fullness, there is a hair filler hidden inside. You can play with the placement and volume and can even add some tendrils hanging down which was a very common detail in Victorian hair.

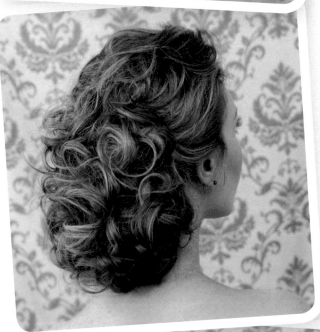

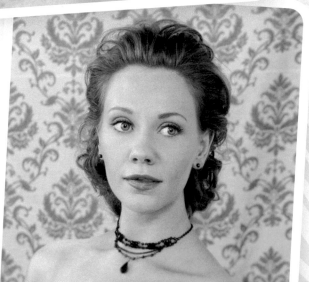

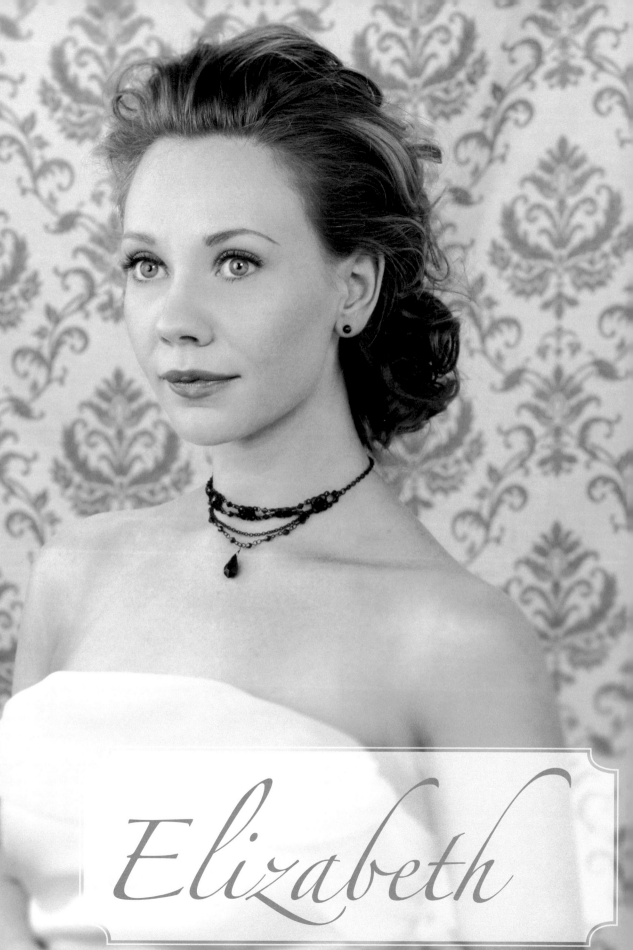

Elizabeth

Supplies

volume spray
thermal hair setting spray
hairspray
pomade

hair dryer
1 - 1/2" tapered curling iron
carbon tail comb
wide tooth comb

grip bob pins
hair clips
hair filler

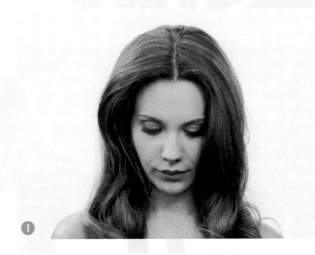

1 Prep the hair using the steps described on page 22. The Elizabeth hairstyle has volume and so the base of the hair should be blow-dried out away from the scalp. Vigorously massage the hair at the scalp while drying to eliminate any unruly growth patterns especially at the front hairline.

Then separate the hair into 2 main sections parted directly down the center of the head.

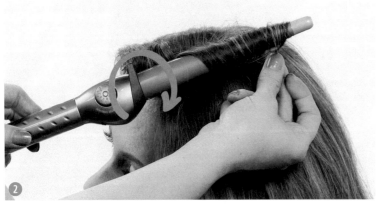

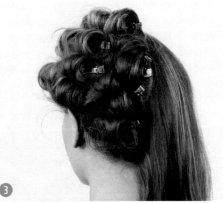

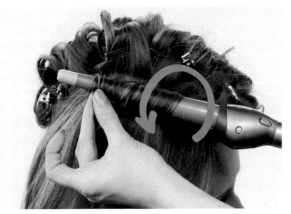

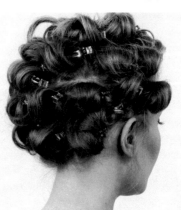

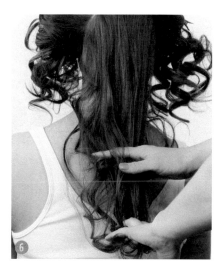

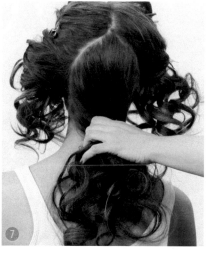

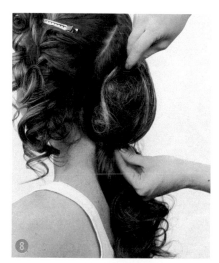

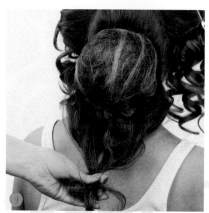

2 On the left section, use the steps described on page 20 to curl the hair with the 1 - 1/2" tapered curling iron in a right wrap pattern. Clip the curls to cool.

3 Curl the entire left side using this method.

4 On the right section, use the steps described on page 21 to curl the hair in a left wrap pattern. Clip the curls.

5 Curl the entire right side using this method.

6 Remove the clips and finger through the curls. Use some pomade on your fingers to aid in separating.

7 Separate a section of hair out that runs from the back of the crown down behind the ears to the nape of the neck. Let this hair lay straight down.

8 Pin a larger, circular hair filler over this section of hair. See page 24 for more about creating a hair filler.

9 Take hold of the ends of the hair below the filler.

10 Bring the ends up over the hair filler.

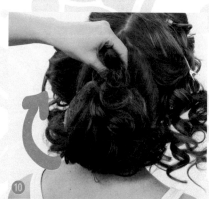

11 Arrange the hair to cover the hair filler and pin in place with grip bob pins.

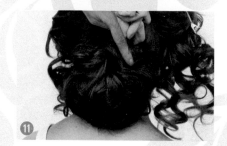

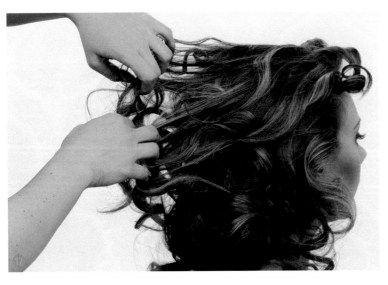
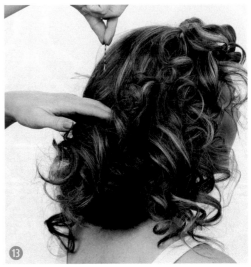

12 Start bringing pieces of hair from the crown back over the hair mass you have started to create in the back. Finger through the curls with some pomade on your fingers to separate out the curls.

13 Pin sections of the hair loosely over the hair filler with grip bob pins.

14 Move to the hair still hanging near the front hairline.

15 Finger through the curls with some pomade on your fingers to separate out the curls and direct them back above the ear.

16 Pin the sides in place and arrange the ends over the back.

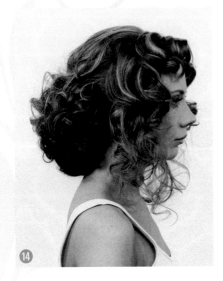
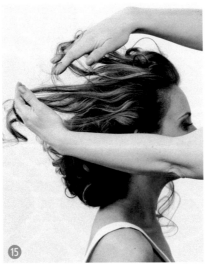
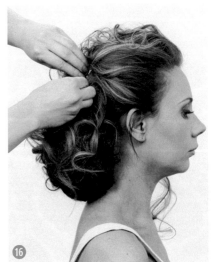

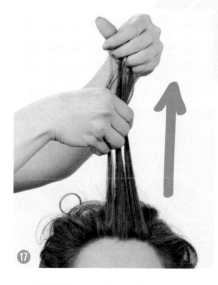
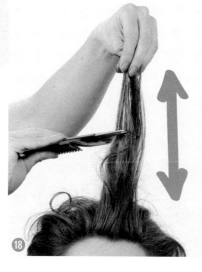
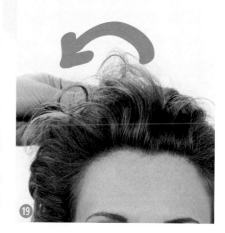

17 With the last few pieces of hair above the forehead, separate the curls for texture.

18 Use a wide tooth comb to lightly tease the hair and add volume to the top of the hairstyle.

19 Bring the last sections back and pin in place loosely.

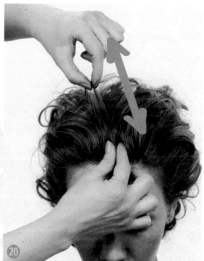

20 Use your fingers to do any final arranging in the front and on the top of the hairstyle. Take special care that the hairstyle from the front has the right balance and form. An important aspect of this style is that, although most of the volume is behind the head, for the purposes of the wedding day pictures, there should also be volume visible from the front.

21 Use grip pins to secure the front section. The best way to do this is to insert the pins from behind and press them forward so they are not visible from the front. Lightly hairspray the style.

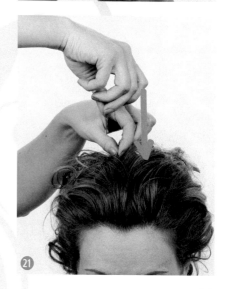

The **Celia** hairstyle draws inspiration from the Gibson Girl illustrations by Charles Dana Gibson in the early 1900s. Characterized as the personification of ideal feminine beauty, the drawings greatly influenced young, fashionable women and the way they wore their hair.

   For this interpretation for an Edwardian inspired wedding, keep the hair full and loose at the top. To keep the face slender looking, taper the hair a little tighter above the ear. The French twist that amasses at the back of the crown is a play on the high bun many Gibson Girls were drawn to have.

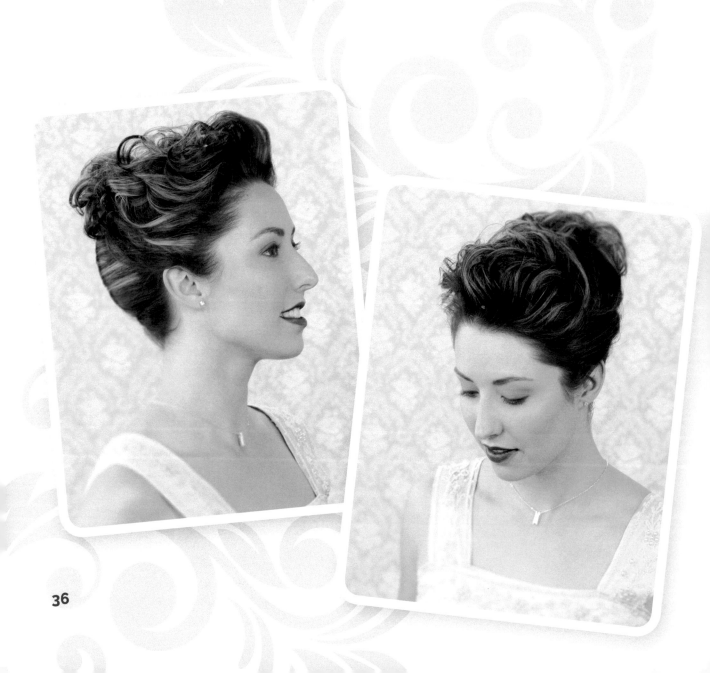

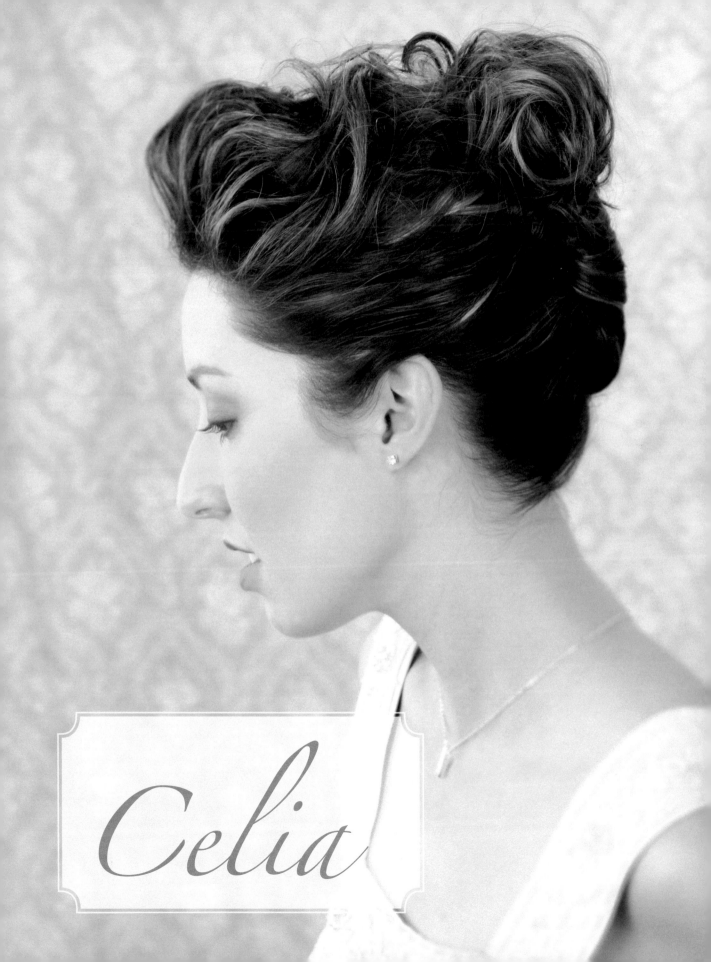

Celia

Supplies

volume spray
thermal hair setting spray
hairspray
pomade
hair dryer

hair dryer diffuser
    attachment
hot rollers
carbon tail comb
wide tooth comb
grip bob pins

ripple hair pins
duckbill clips
hair filler
2 ¾" plastic craft needle
lightweight monofilament

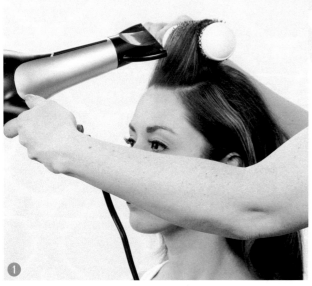

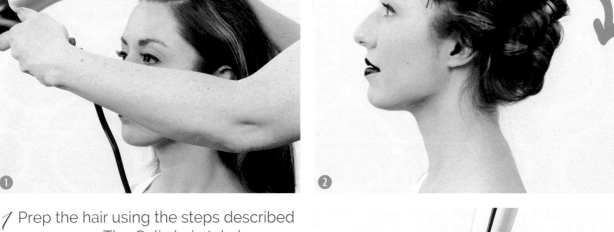

1 Prep the hair using the steps described on page 22. The Celia hairstyle has volume and so the base of the hair should be blow-dried out away from the scalp. Vigorously massage the hair at the scalp while you blow-dry to eliminate any unruly growth patterns especially at the front hairline.

2 Set the entire head in small hot rollers in a bricklay pattern. See page 13 for tips on hot rollers.

3 Use a hair dryer with diffuser attachment on high heat to add extra setting power to the curlers.

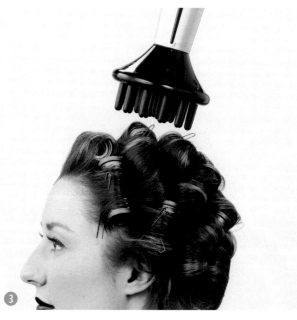

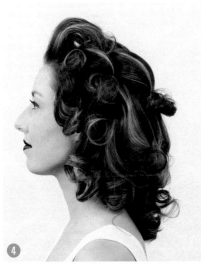

4 Remove the curlers after they have cooled completely.

5 Separate the hair in to 2 sections. One section includes the hair at the back of the crown, down behind the ears, and to the nape of the neck. The other section is everything else at the front hairline back to the ears.

6 The back section of hair is going to be styled into a French twist. Start by brushing all of the hair in this section to the right and hold it tightly. Insert large grip pins criss-crossing to hold the hair flat against the scalp.

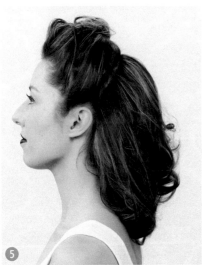

7 For extra hold and control, I created a small, long, flat hair filler to be pinned over the large grip pins. This will help give stability to the style. See page 24 for more about creating a hair filler.

8 The last step for the back section is to twist and fold the ends of the hair over the hair filler and insert grip pins horizontally through the crease to lock the twist to the hair filler underneath. The ends of the hair that should now be at the top of the twist can be left alone for now. They will be used later on.

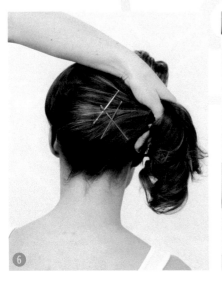

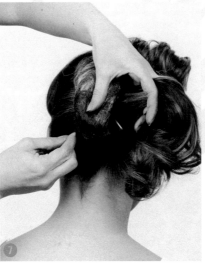

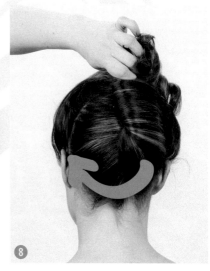

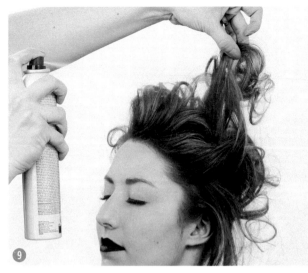

9 Move on to the front section. Finger through the curls and loosely spray them with a lightweight hairspray to add texture.

Be sure to do this gently. There should be a lot of volume at the top of this hairstyle to mimic the volume of a classic Gibson Girl hairstyle. If the hair at the top of the style is too flat against the scalp, it loses the effect.

10 Use a wide tooth comb or hair pick to gently tease texture and volume into the section.

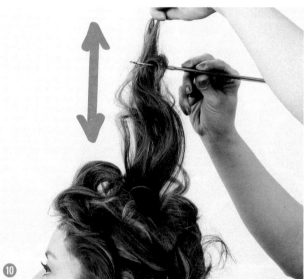

11 Direct the curls back toward the top of the French twist gently with your fingers. Take care that you still have the volume on top of the head. The hair should sit 2-3 inches above the top of the head.

12 To finish this hairstyle, hair sewing is going to be used. The purpose is to secure the style and its curls as best as possible without compromising the loose, easy feel of the form. See page 26 for more information about hair sewing.

Begin at the front, an inch or so behind the hairline. Secure the monofilament in a hidden section of the hair. Sew a line across using large stitches from one ear up and over to the other ear. Direct the sewing deeper at the scalp as opposed to the higher level of the outer form.

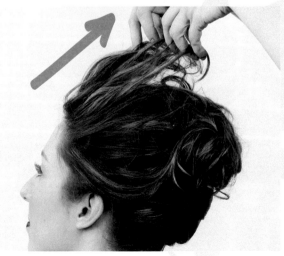

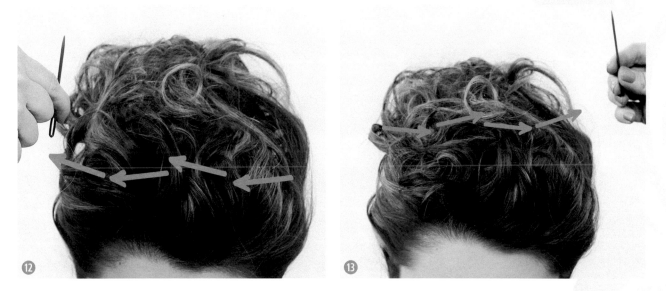

13 Sew another line about an inch back from the first across to the other side. Continue these lines until you reach the top of the French twist. Secure the end of the monofilament knotting it to the hair so it does not unravel.

14 Now that the top section is secure, you can refine the shape at the top. Use your fingers to gently tug the hair into the desired form and create the texture.

15 Tug the front of the hairline to achieve the desired volume.

16 Use a tail comb to form the area around the top of the French twist and use grip bob pins to secure the style. Lightly hairspray the hair.

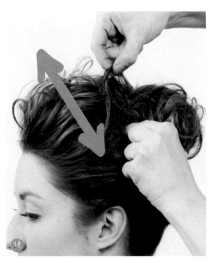
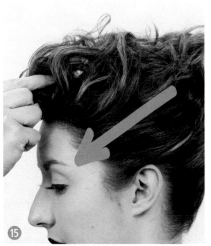
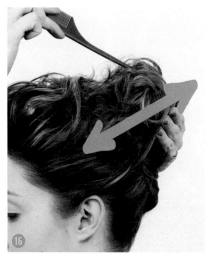

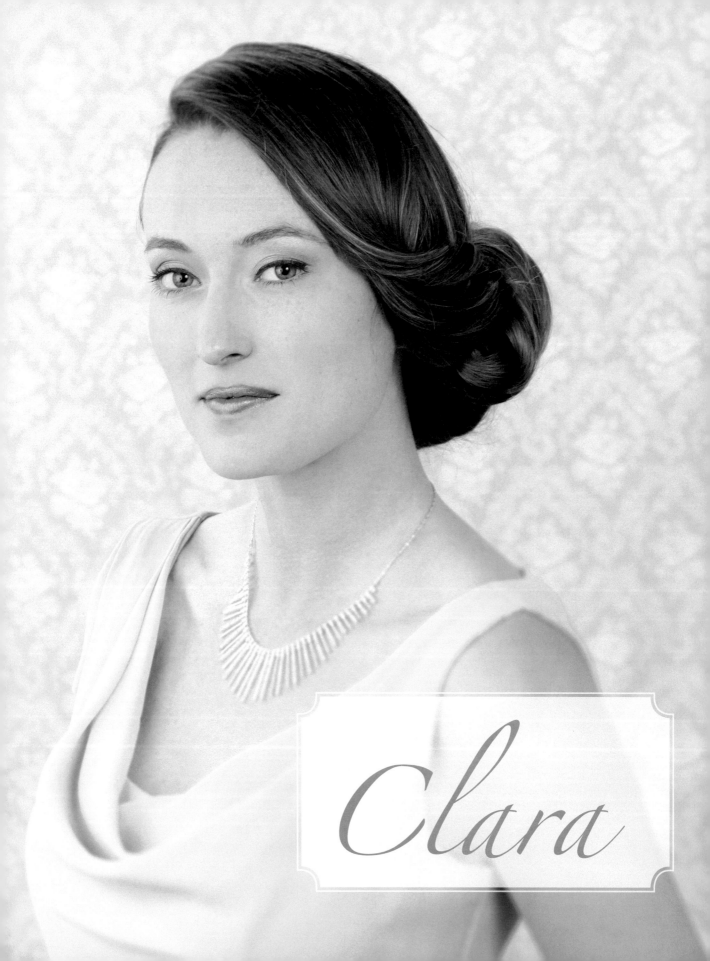

Clara

The silhouette of the **Clara** hairstyle is asymmetric. On the right side it is tight against the head. On the left, it is full and loose.

Although the silhouette is not the same as a typical Edwardian hairstyle, the Clara is still categorized with the early 1900s hairstyles because of the techniques used. Edwardian women set their very long hair in curls and then pinned it up in random series of loose twists and buns. This same idea can be used in many different silhouettes to create a soft bodied up-do.

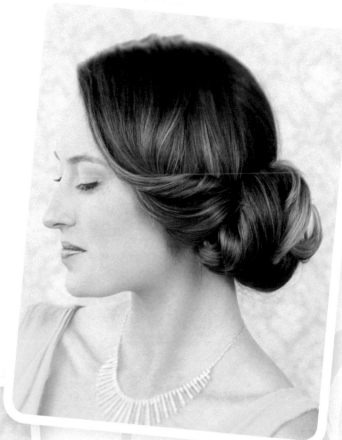

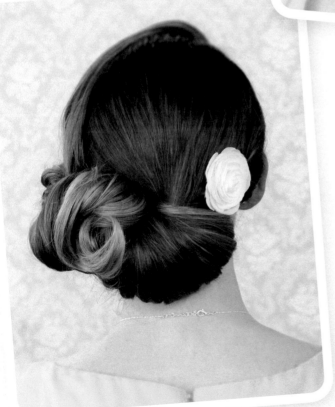

Supplies

thermal hair setting spray
hairspray
pomade
1" curling iron

carbon tail comb
loop and tail styling tool
grip bob pins
ripple hair pins

duckbill clips
hair clips
rubber bands (small and large)
hair filler

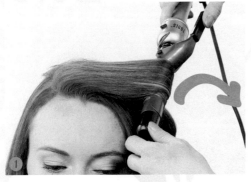

1 Prep the hair using the steps described on page 22 for setting product into the hair. This hairstyle has a severe side part on the right, so use the steps described on page 23 to move the natural part over so that it lies above the outer corner of the right eyebrow.

2 Curl all of the hair with a 1" curling iron. Pin the curls with hair clips and allow them to cool before you begin.

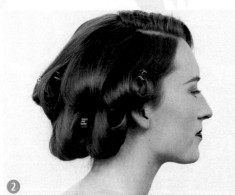

3 Using a tail comb, create an upside down C-shape section from the part and down and around behind the ear on the right side of the head. Clip back the rest of the hair to keep it out of the way. Comb the hair section straight down. Use grip pins in a criss-cross fashion to pin the hair tight against the scalp. Keep the pins focused toward the back.

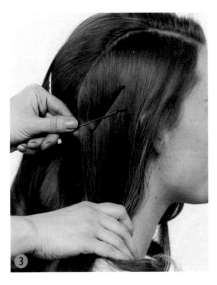
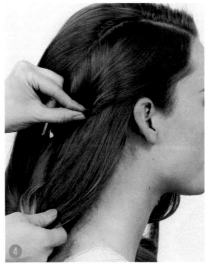
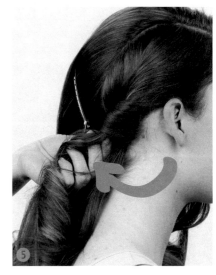

4 Because the pins were focused toward the back of the C-shape section, there should be some hair free at the hairline above the ear. Bring this section back to expose the ear and pin it tightly over the existing grip pins.

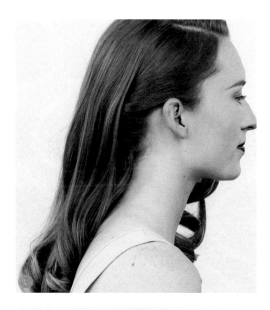

5 Now take this entire hair section you have been working with made by the C-shape sectioning and twist it up to expose the right side of the neck and grip pin it in place.

6 Release the rest of the hair that was clipped out of the way in step 3.

7 The next section of hair to work with encompasses the C-shape piece below the part that we just worked with. It also includes the hair at the back of the head that reaches from the back of the crown down behind the ears and to the nape of the neck. All of this hair is brushed into a low ponytail. The ponytail should sit half way between the occipital bone and the nape of the neck, almost in line with the center of the ears. Use the method described on page 27 to create a secure ponytail.

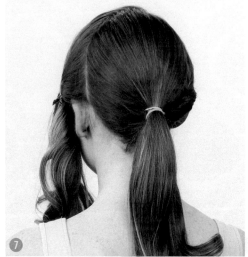

8 This step requires a dense hair filler in a cylindrical shape that is just long enough to stretch from behind the ear of one side, down to the nape of the neck, and over and up to behind the other ear. In this scenario, I used a hair padding from Sharon Blain Education that is perfect for this hairstyle. See the resource section in the back of the book.

Pin the filler in a horseshoe shape. The pins should be arranged so that they hold the filler to the scalp, but be careful that the pins do not hinder the free movement of the hair in the ponytail for later in the hairstyle. The lower portion of the filler presses the ponytail tight against neck

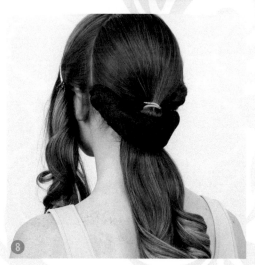

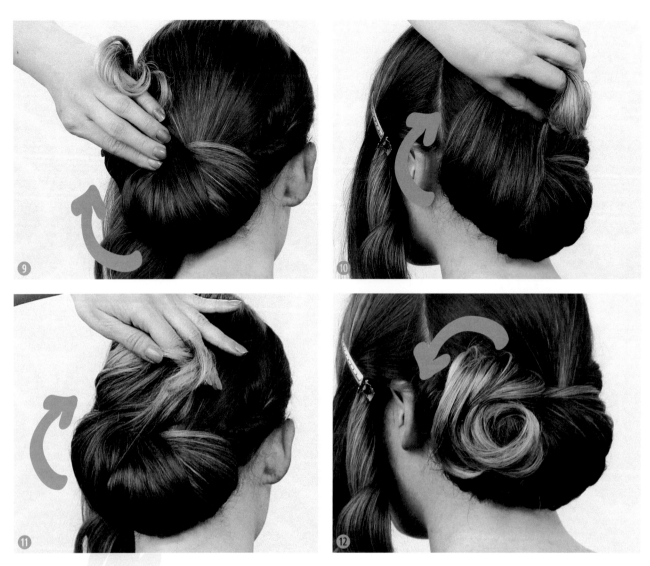

9 Start the next few steps with separating the ponytail into 2 pieces. Starting with the right piece, bring it up and over the hair filler to cover a portion of it. It helps to use the ripple pins to hold the hair in place while you manipulate it into the best position. See page 28 for information on using ripple pins this way.

10 Bring the left section of the ponytail up over the left of the hair filler.

11 Spread the hair so that the entire hair filler is covered. Grip pin everything in place.

12 Arrange the ends of the hair into a pin curl.

13 You have one area of hair left to work with. It includes the hair to the left from the part down to the ear. Separate this last section into 3 long sections with the parts running from the part of the right eyebrow and down to the lower left hairline.

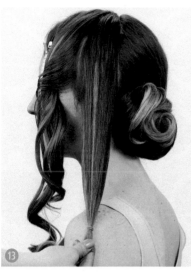

13 With the piece of hair to the rear, closest to the chignon you just made, comb the hair down toward the shoulder. Attach a small rubber band tightly around the ends of the hair to hold them together.

14 Rotate the ends in an arch up and back toward the chignon. Use a couple grip bob pins, attach them to the rubber band and then pin this piece into the hair filler inside the chignon.

15 Move on to the next piece of hair and repeat the steps of attaching a small rubber band tightly around the ends of the hair to hold them together.

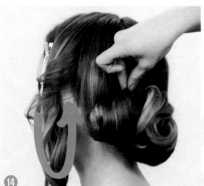

16 Rotate the ends in an arch up and back toward the piece from before. Use a couple grip bob pins, attach them to the rubber band and then pin this piece to secure it.

17 With the last piece toward the front, attach the same small rubber band tightly to the ends.

18 Rotate the ends in an arch up and back. Use a tail loop tool to weave the ends through the piece behind it. Hide and grip pin the ends of this piece to secure it.

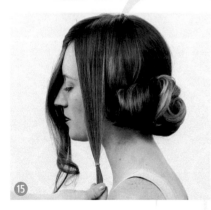

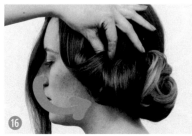

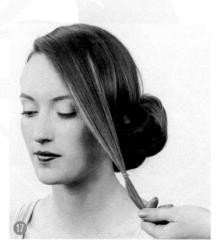

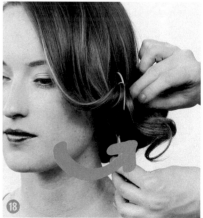

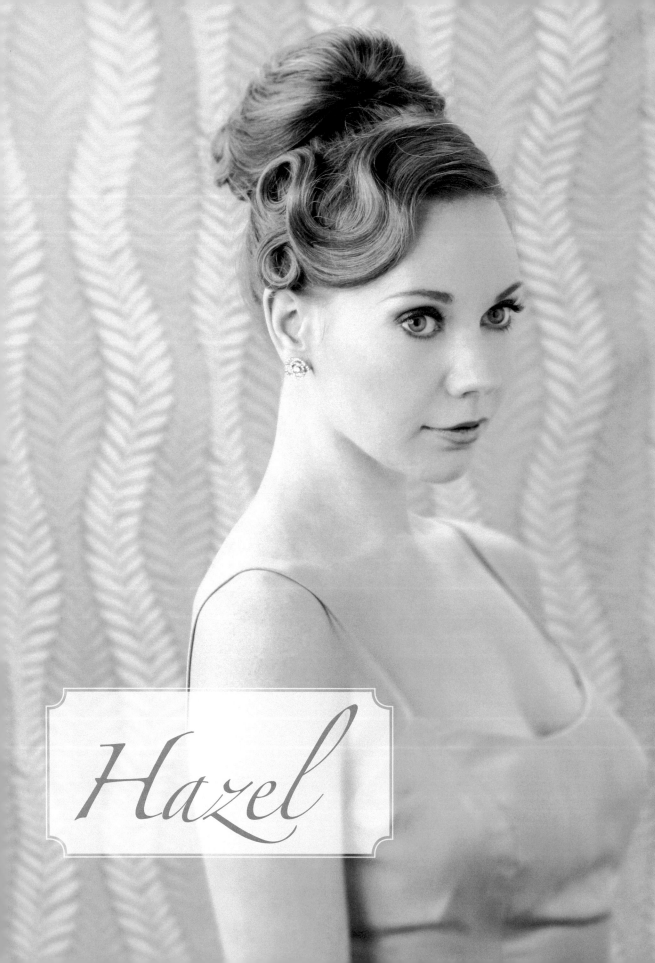

Hazel

The focal point of the **Hazel** hairstyle, the deep wave of the fringe, is inspired by contemporary interpretations of the Jazz Age and the Great Gatsby lifestyle. Using modern hairstyling techniques like curling irons to create the finger wave effect makes the style a little softer and delicate.

The silhouette of the 1920s was often face framing and low by the nape of the neck and chin. The faux bob is a way to copy this silhouette, but for the Hazel hairstyle, the high bun at the crown adds a fresh perspective on the inspiration. Consider switching the silhouette of the back of any Jazz Age hairstyle when you are working with a large group and need some variation between them.

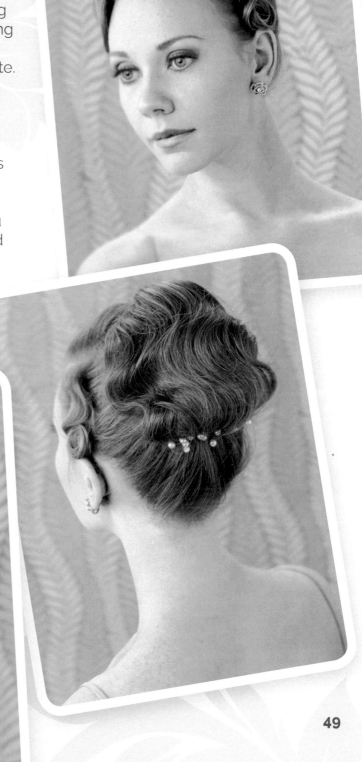

49

Supplies

thermal hair setting spray	¾" curling iron	duckbill clips
hairspray	¾ - ½" tapered curling iron	hair clips
pomade	carbon tail comb	large rubber bands
hair dryer	natural bristle grooming brush	hair net with elastic
hair dryer diffuser	grip bob pins	playing cards
attachment	ripple hair pins	

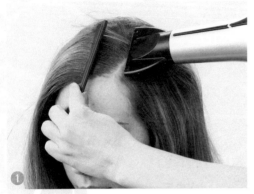

1 Prep using the steps described on page 22 for setting product into the hair. Use the steps described on page 23 to set the part over so that it lies above the outer corner of the left eyebrow.

2 There are 3 main sections to this style. Create 2 small sections, one on either side of the part. The section above the part should be 2 times wider than the section below the part.

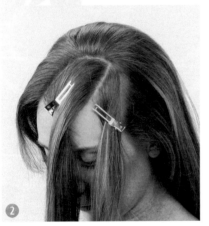
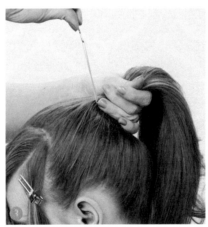
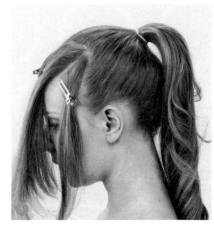

3 Bring the entire rest of the hair into a high ponytail above the occipital bone.

4 Use the steps described on page 27 to secure the ponytail tightly.

5 Start with the small section of hair to the left of the part and the ¾" curling iron,

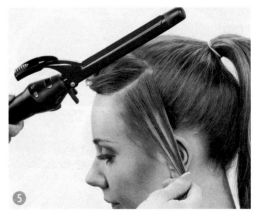

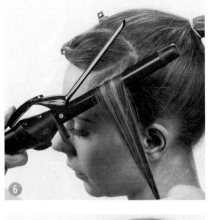

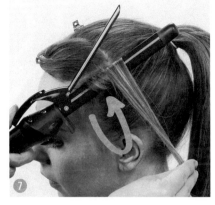

6 Hold the section of hair in your right hand. Hold the curling iron in your left hand close to the scalp with out touching it. Use the wrapping technique the same as the tapered wand wrap technique described on page 20.

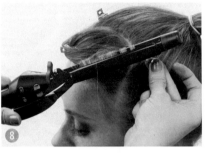

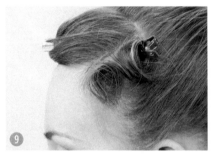

7 Wrap the hair section over the top of the wand and under to the right.

8 With each wrap around the curling iron, the hair moves to the right along the wand and does not overlap the previous wrap around.

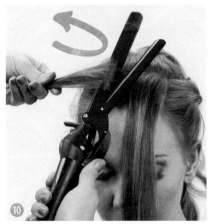

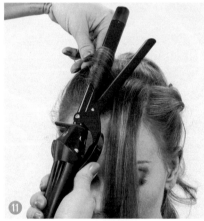

9 Clip the curl to cool.

10 On the right section, separate a 1 inch section.

11 Repeat the previous steps to curl the hair, but holding the curling iron in your right hand, the hair in your left, and wrap the hair to the left down the curling iron wand.

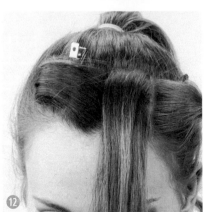

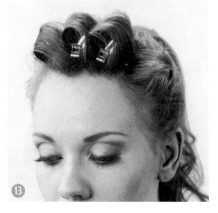

12 Clip the curl to cool.

13 Create 3 curls above the forehead.

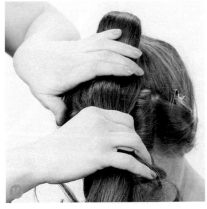
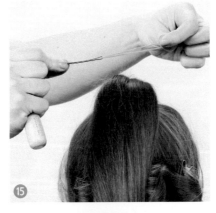
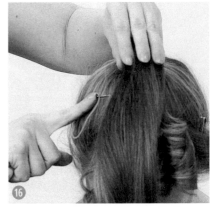

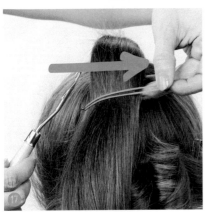
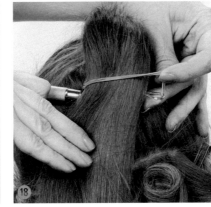
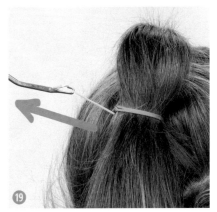

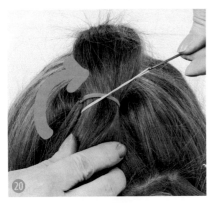

Steps 14-21 below describe the method for creating the spray effect at the front of the bun of this hairstyle.

14 Take entire ponytail and bring it over the top of the head.

15 Attach a grip pin to a large rubber band.

16 Attach the pin horizontally to the hair under the ponytail about an inch forward from the base.

17 Wrap the rubber band over the top of the ponytail.

18 Weave the latch hook through the hair at the scalp, in front of the grip pin and grab hold of the rubber band.

19 Pull the rubber band back through the hair at the scalp.

20 Wrap the rubber band one more time over the ponytail.

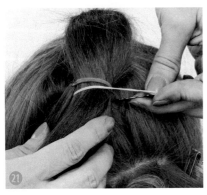

21 Use a grip pin to secure the rubber band end under the ponytail close to the first grip pin.

22 Separate about 2/3 of the hair out of the ponytail. This section is going to be used to create a hair filler.

23 Back brush this section and bring it back behind the head. Smooth the hair with the brush for a cleaner appearance.

24 Wrap a hair net with elastic around the hair mass.

25 Bring the hairnet under.

26 Arrange the hair mass into a bun form and pin the hairnet to the scalp.

27 With all of this, you should have a large, round, bun shaped hair filler.

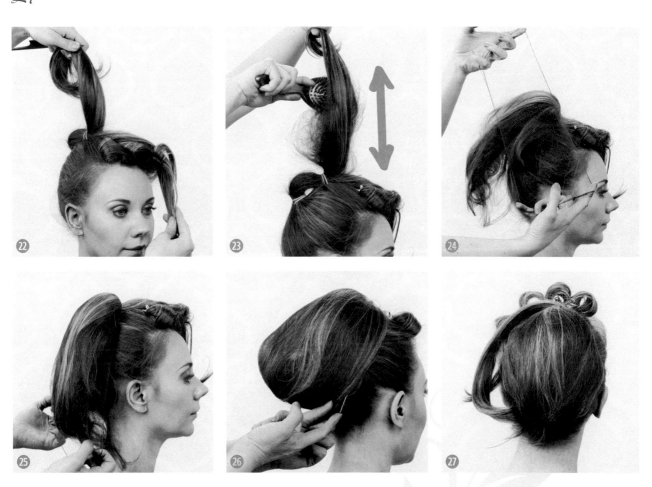

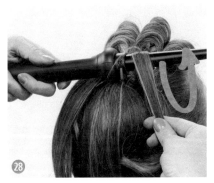

28 You still have a small section left from the ponytail that will now be curled. Separate this section into 5 or 6 pieces. Use the ¾ - ½" tapered curling iron. These pieces will be combed into deep waves and the smaller tapered curling iron is best for this.

29 Curl each piece using the right wrap pattern described on page 20. It is important that these curls are all created uniformly.

30 Use caution not to burn your fingers.

31 Clip the curls to cool.

32 Remove the hair clips and separate out a section. You are going to comb the curls out in pieces, not all at once.

33 Comb out and back-comb the section to start spreading the wave and locking the hairs together.

34 Bring the section over the left side of the hair filler created on the previous page.

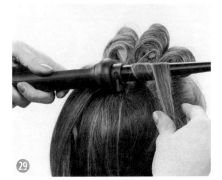

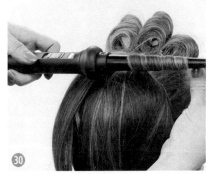

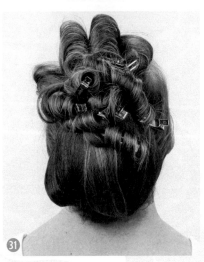

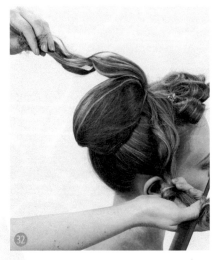

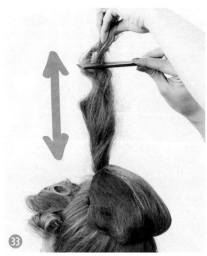

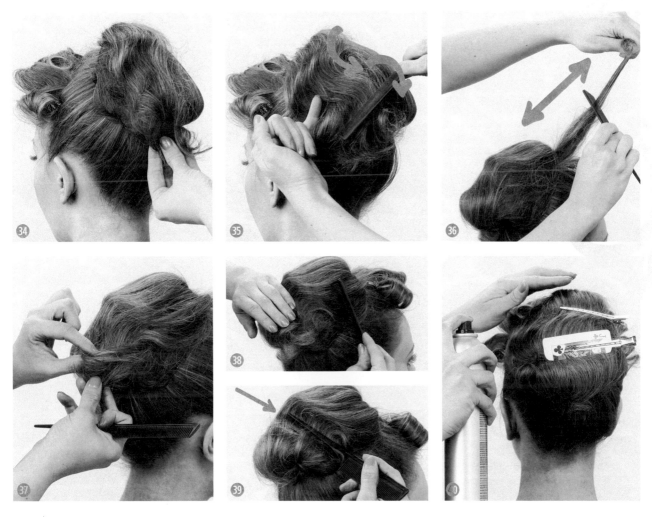

35 Gently comb over in a wave pattern in small controled strokes to smooth the visible side of the wave.

36 Take another section of curls in your hand and repeat the steps. Comb out and back-comb to spread the wave and lock the hairs together.

37 Bring the section over the right side of the hair filler. Continue these steps until the entire hair filler is covered.

38 Manipulate the waves to line up with each other around the entire hair mass.

39 Use the tail of the comb to press the waves deeper.

40 Clip the deepest parts of the waves with duckbill clips to enhance the shape. Use pieces of playing cards between the clips and the hair to avoid marks. Spray with a lightweight hairspray.

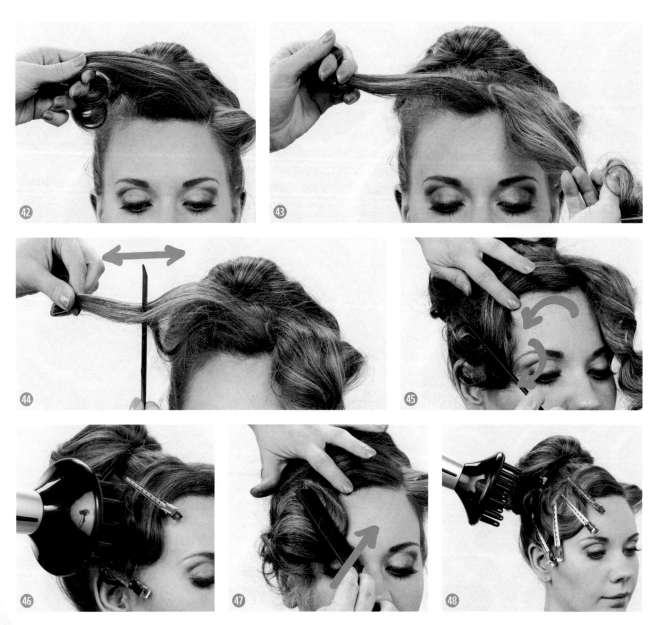

42 Remove the hair clips from the section of hair above the part.

43 Separate it into 2 sections.

44 Using the lower section, comb out and back-comb the section to start spreading the wave and locking the hairs together.

45 Comb the hair against the right side of the head to start forming it into a wave. Comb forward and back in a wave pattern to guide and manipulate and hold each portion of the wave against the scalp as you comb.

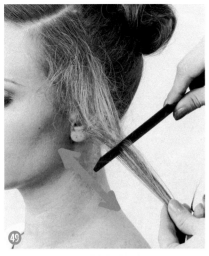

46 Clip the waves with duckbill clips to hold the shape. Heat the wave up with the hair dryer diffuser attachment and then allow it to cool to help set the wave.

47 Continue these steps on the second piece, waving the hair into its form.

48 Use duckbill clips to hold the form and heat the wave up with the hair dryer diffuser attachment and then allow it to cool to help set the wave.

49 With the last piece of hair to the left of the part, comb out and back-comb the section to start spreading the wave and locking the hairs together.

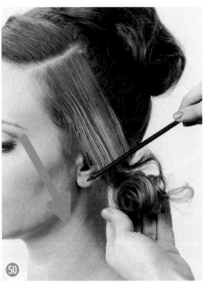

50 Smooth with a comb.

51 Hold the end of the curl in your left hand.

52 Use your right hand to press a wave form against the scalp. Bring the end up into a pin curl.

53 Clip with duckbill clips to hold the shape. Heat the wave up with the hair dryer diffuser attachment and then allow it to cool to help set the wave.

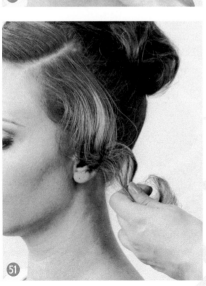

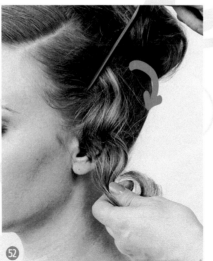

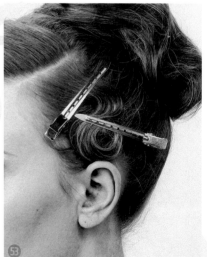

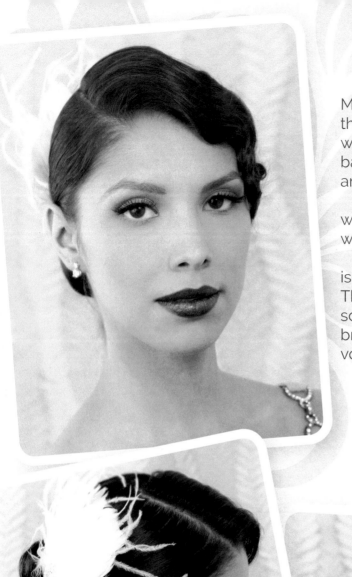

Many images of hairstyle silhouettes from the Jazz Age give the impression that most women had their hair cropped short in the back. A lot of women in fact had long hair and pinned it up to be fashionable.

The **Rose** hairstyle combines this idea with a finger wave look in the front created with a curling iron.

Note in the steps, the wave at the front is created using a very thin slices of hair. This helps keep the wave close to the scalp and makes it easier to control when brushing it out. If you would like more volume on top, use more hair in steps 4-6.

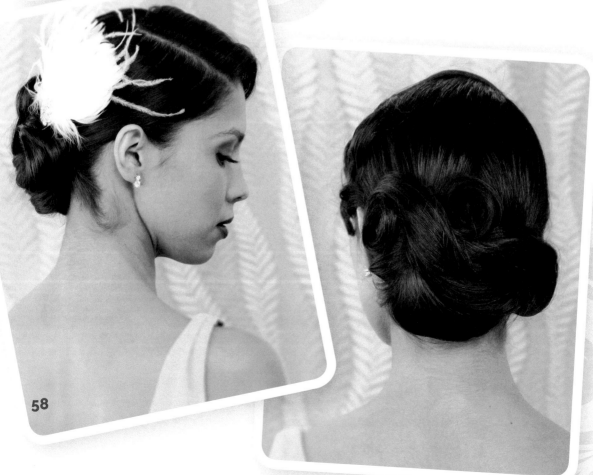

58

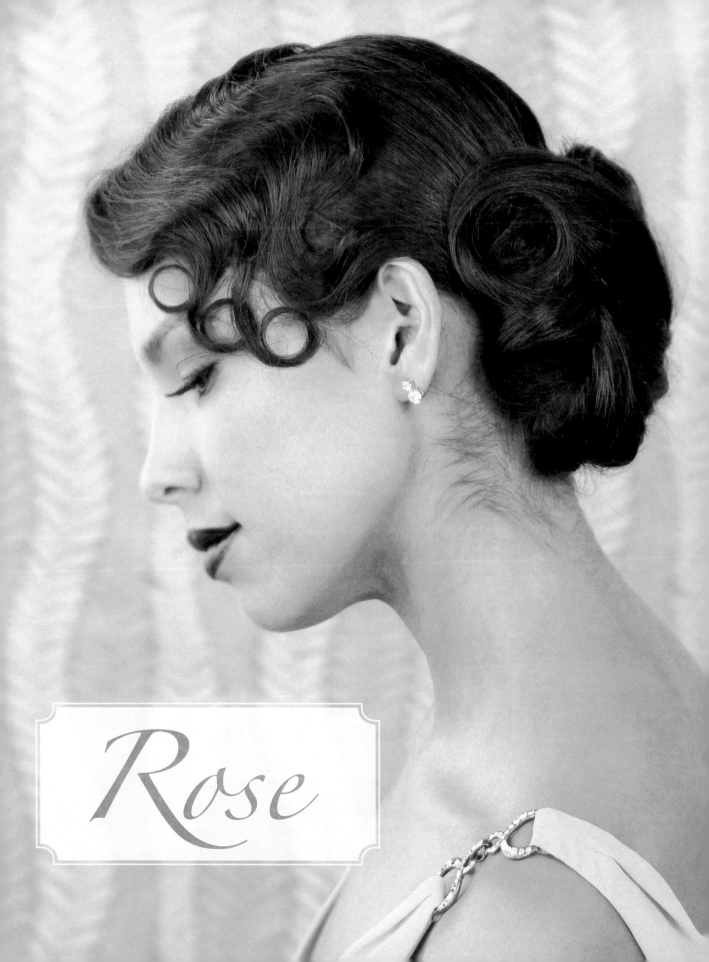

Rose

Supplies

thermal hair setting spray
hairspray
pomade
hair dryer
hair dryer diffuser
    attachment

½" curling iron
1" curling iron
carbon tail comb
styling brush
grip bob pins

ripple hair pins
duckbill clips
hair clips
small rubber bands
playing cards

1 Prep using the steps described on page 22 for setting product into the hair. Use the steps described on page 23 to set the part over so that it lies above the outer corner of the right eyebrow.

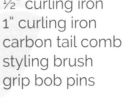

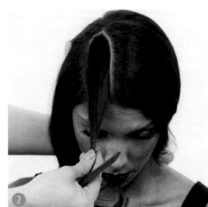

2 There are 2 main sections to this hairstyle. One section stretches from the part and 1 inch to the left. It then stretches back about 4 inches to the back of the crown. The other section is the entire rest of the hair.

3 Curl the larger section with the 1" curling iron.

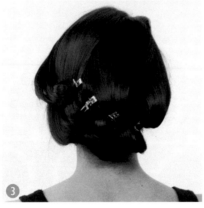

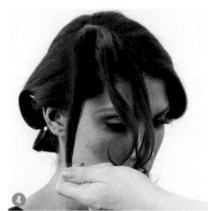

4 Separate the smaller section into 3 long, diagonal sections.

5 Curl these 3 pieces with the ½" curling iron into tight curls.

6 Clip the curls to cool.

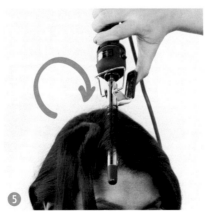

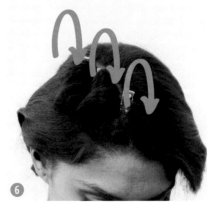

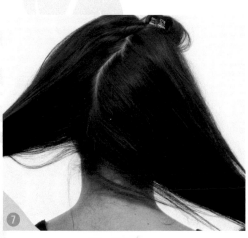

7 Move to the larger section. Part it diagonally from the left side of the base of the neck, up to the right, and connect with the back of the curls at the top of the head.

8 With the section on the right, create a tight, low ponytail. Then do the same with the hair on the left. Parting and creating the ponytails this way helps to hide any visible parting in the back.

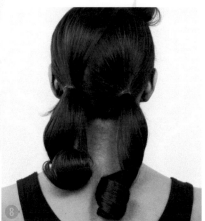
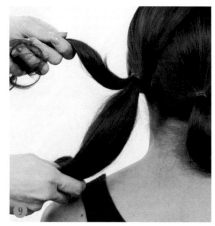
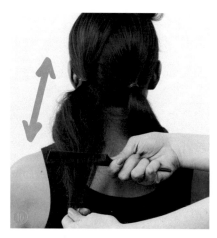

9 Separate the left ponytail in 2 sections.

10 Back-comb deeply into one section to lock the hairs together. Extra back-combing is recommended to lock the hair for more secure hold in the next steps.

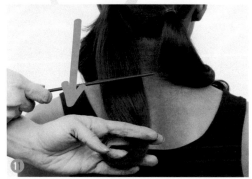

11 Smooth the visible side with a comb.

12 Now rotate, twist, and manipulate the piece to cover the base of the ponytail. Play with the angle and configuration. Grip pin the hair to the hair underneath to secure it.

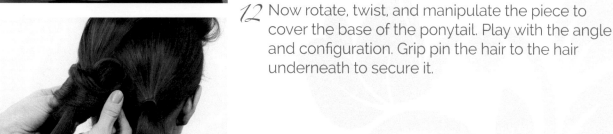

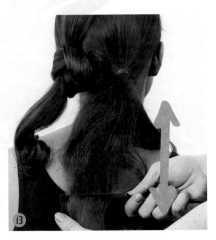 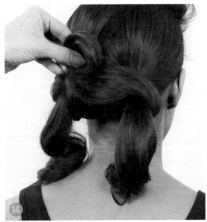 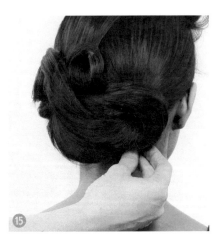

13 Use the same steps on the ponytail on the right. Separate it in 2 sections. Back-comb deeply into one piece to spread and lock the hairs together. Extra back-combing is recommended. Smooth the visible side with a comb.

14 Now rotate, twist, and manipulate the piece to cover the base of the ponytail. Play with the angle and configuration. Grip pin the hair to the scalp hair underneath to secure it.

15 There are now 2 pieces of hair left, one on either side. Manipulate these pieces the same way. Back-comb deeply to spread the wave and lock the hairs together and smooth the visible side. Then rotate, twist, and manipulate the piece to create waves. Hide grip bob pins in the style to secure it.

16 Remove the hair clips from the small curls at the top of the head. Brush out and back-comb the hair to spread the wave and locking the hairs together.

17 Comb the hair down the left side of the head to start forming it into a wave.

18 Move the comb forward and back in a wave pattern to guide and manipulate and hold each portion of the wave against the scalp as you comb.

19 Press the comb's teeth gently into the scalp and then up toward the top of the head to help define the ridge of the wave.

20 Clip the deepest parts of the waves with duckbill clips to enhance the shape. Use pieces of playing cards between the clips and the hair to avoid marks.

21 When you have combed to above the ear, start separating the ends into tiny curls. Use a little pomade on your fingers to define the curls and add shine.

22 Manipulate the curls to lay flat against the hairline in spit curl fashion. To help stick the curls to the face, spray some hairspray directly on the skin and then press the curl onto the spot of hairspray. Use duckbill clips to hold things in place and heat the area with the hair dryer set high with the diffuser attachment to help set the style.

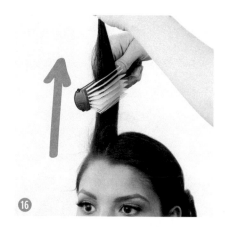

16

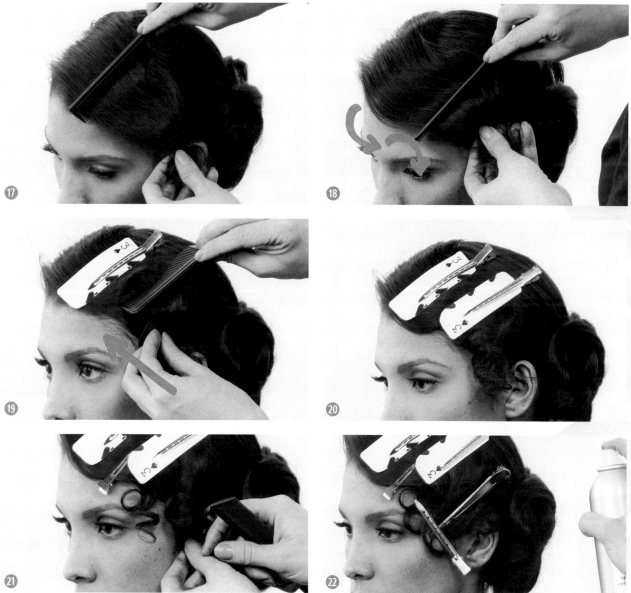

17

18

19

20

21

22

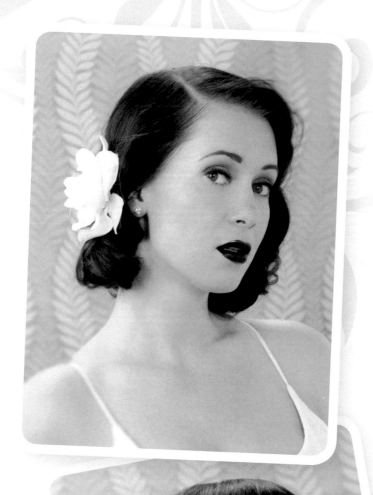

The silhouette of the **Victoria** hairstyle is inspired by the 1920s style that followed the shape of the head closely. Women either cut their hair in a shingled bob or they pinned their hair tight at the nape of the neck. The result was a style that could be worn well under a cloche hat, the hat of any fashionable woman of the day.

The texture is also important to this hairstyle. Instead of sleek, uniform finger waves, the waves are loose and soft.

It is designed as an up-do, but the loose waves and lack of a specific focal point adds a casualness to the style that makes it great for a day event.

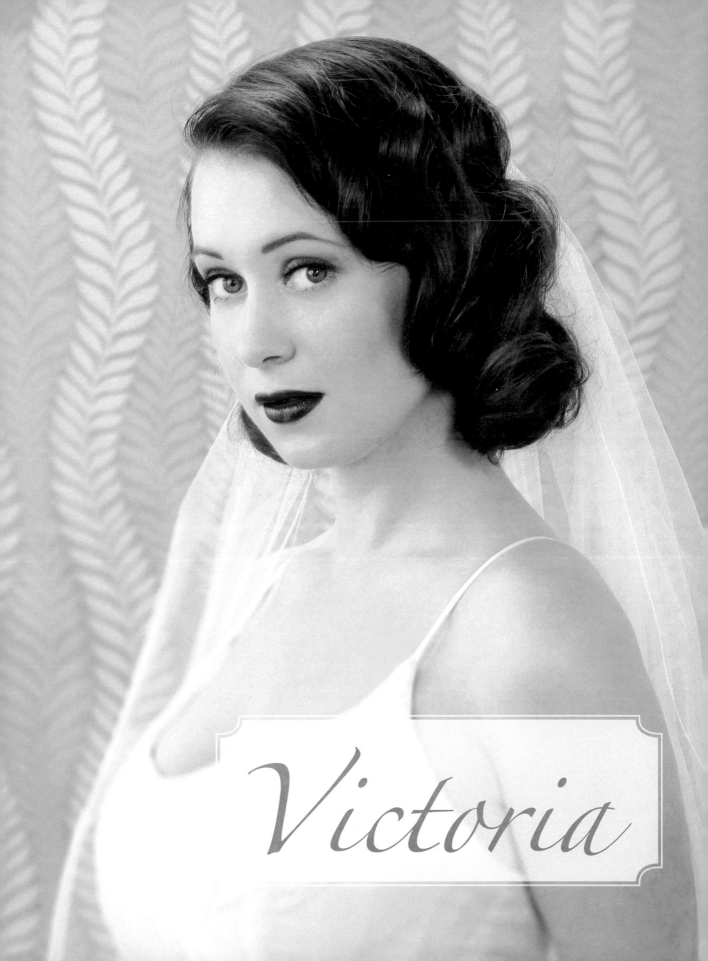

Victoria

Supplies

thermal hair setting spray	1 - ½" tapered curling iron	ripple hair pins
hairspray	carbon tail comb	hair clips
pomade	wide tooth comb	2 ¾" plastic craft needle
hair dryer	grip bob pins	lightweight monofilament

1 Prep using the steps described on page 22 for setting product into the hair and adding volume to the hairstyle. Use the steps described on page 23 to set the part over so that it lies above the outer corner of the right eyebrow.

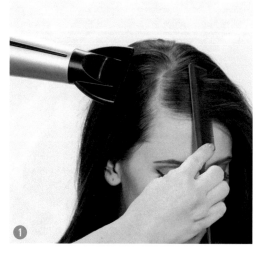

2 Before curling, separate the hair into 2 sections. The first section is on the right side of the head. Create a c-shape that curves around from the back of the part.

3 Use the steps described on page 21 to curl the hair in this first section in a left wrap pattern. Use the 1 - ½" tapered curling iron and 1x1 inch sections of hair.

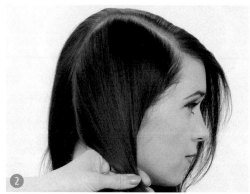

4 Use caution not to burn your fingers.

5 Clip the curls to cool.

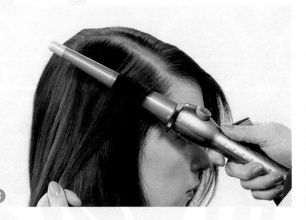

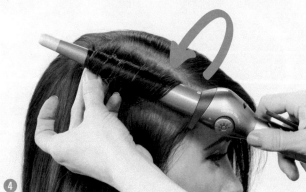

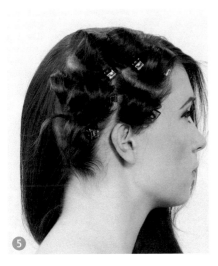
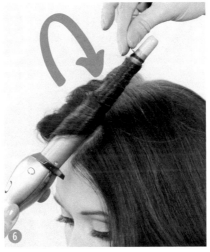
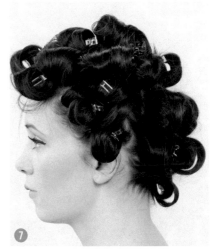

6 Curl the rest of the hair on the entire head using the right wrap pattern described on page 20 using 1x1" sections of hair.

7 Clip the hair to cool.

8 Once the hair has finished cooling, use a hair pick to loosely comb out the curls one row at a time starting from the bottom.

9 On the right side, comb the hair directly down toward the shoulder.

10 On the left, leave the final top row of curls to the left of the part alone for now. Comb out the left side one row of curls at a time directly down toward the shoulder.

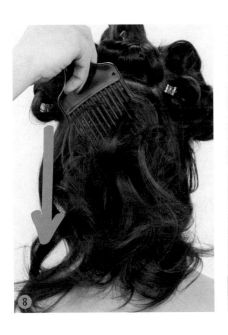
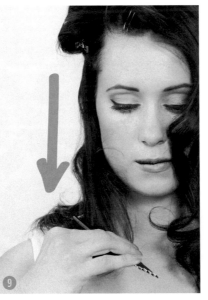
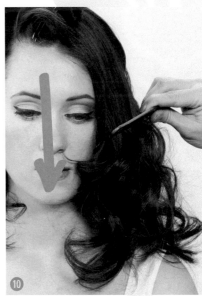

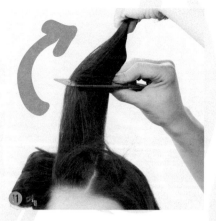
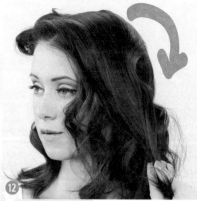
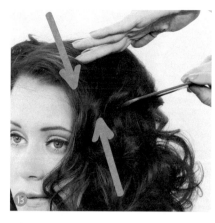

Because the tapered curling iron does such a good job of producing a wave, you will already see the soft, vintage waves taking shape.

11 Remove the clips from the final top row of curls to the left of the part. Comb the entire piece together in one mass straight up from the scalp to add some lift to the top.

12 Allow this piece to fold over gently to the left side.

13 Using your hand and a comb, gently massage and press the ridge and wave at the edge of the crown to help define it more.

14 Now hair sewing is going to be used to secure the style, but also it will aid in forming the loose shape of the waves in this hairstyle. See the steps described on page 26 to learn more about sewing. Thread a craft needle with monofilament and knot the end to the hair.

15 Start a line to "sew" that will run just below the first ridge at the top wave that runs around the crown of the head. The purpose of this step is to secure the hair and keep it tight to the scalp.

16 Continue around the head in a horizontal line. Knot the ends of the monofilament to the hair to keep it from unraveling.

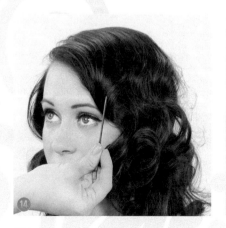
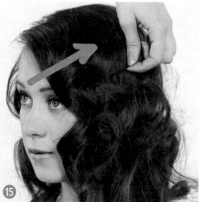
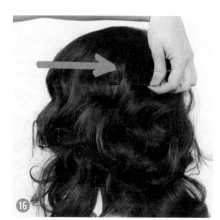

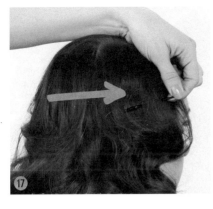
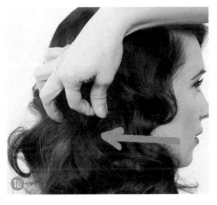
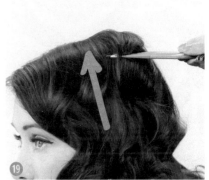

17 Start a new piece of monofilament to sew with. Begin a new sewing line about 1 ½ inches below the first row. Continue to sew around the head in a horizontal line.

18 Sew one last horizontal row below the second. This line should run from just above the ear and around to just above the other ear.

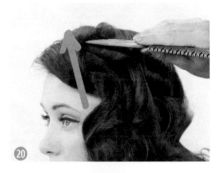

19 Using a hair pick, gently press volume into the top portion of the hairstyle. This will affect the style in 2 ways. First, it adds volume at the crown. Second, this manipulation helps enhance the wave. Because you are pressing up, the hair is being gently tugged up through the secure sewing line. When you release it, gravity will bring the hair down, define the ridge even more, and enhance the depth in the wave.

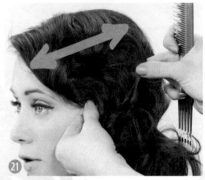

20 Continue to press and manipulate gently through the hairstyle for volume.

21 Use your fingers to further manipulate the shape. Tug gently where needed to bring out the texture.

22 Spray with a lightweight hairspray.

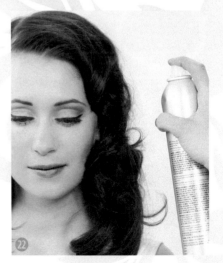

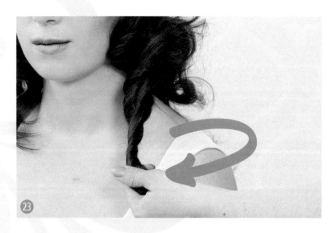
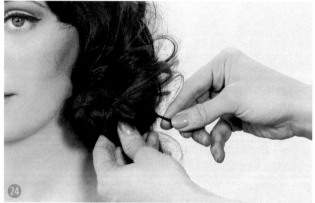

23 Now that the crown and interior have been shaped, it is time to secure the bottom into a faux bob that holds tight again the neckline. Working in small sections, twist the ends of the hair hanging down.

24 Twist the ends up into themselves and use the monofilament to sew the piece to secure it. A good technique to use here is to thread the needle through in varying directions to make sure all of the hair is confined.

25 Tug tight enough to keep everything together.

26 Work around the back of the neck with the same method. Twist the ends of the hair hanging down up into themselves and use the monofilament to sew the pieces secure. Keep the shape close to the neckline to mimic the close bob of the 1920s.

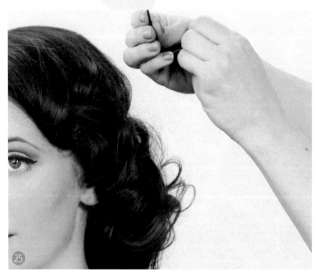
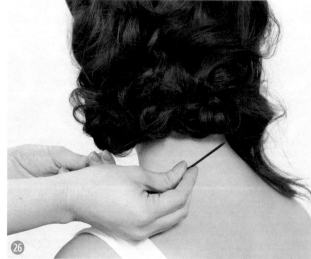

27 Continue to the opposite side of the hairstyle, sewing the ends into twisted pin curl shapes and vary the direction of the sewing needle to secure all of the ends.

28 Try not to use only one piece of monofilament for this lower section. A lot of weight is being placed in this area and for security it is best to have 2-3 different strands running through the lower section for security in case a piece breaks. It is better to overdo it for a hairstyle on such an important day.

29 It is also a good idea to take one last piece of monofilament and sew through to refine any areas that need it. Knot all monofilament ends to the hair to keep them from unraveling.

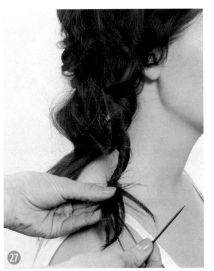
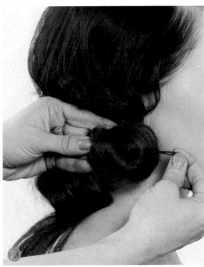
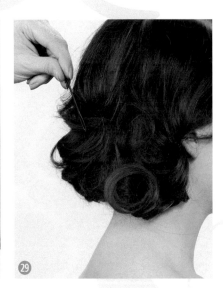

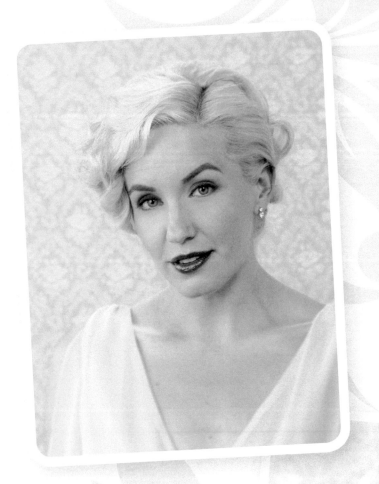

The **Joan** hairstyle is inspired by many film actresses of the 1930s. For example, Norma Shearer wore a mixture of tight and loose waves angled differently from each other to create very interesting geometric shapes in the silhouette. Different from the waves of the 1910s and 1920s which emphasized symmetry and repetition, in the 1930s the form of the interior of the hairstyle under the waves took different shapes.

   This hairstyle works better on fine or medium hair textures with layers. Note the techniques in the following steps used to hide the ends in the interior of the hairstyle. Hiding the ends makes for a cleaner finish.

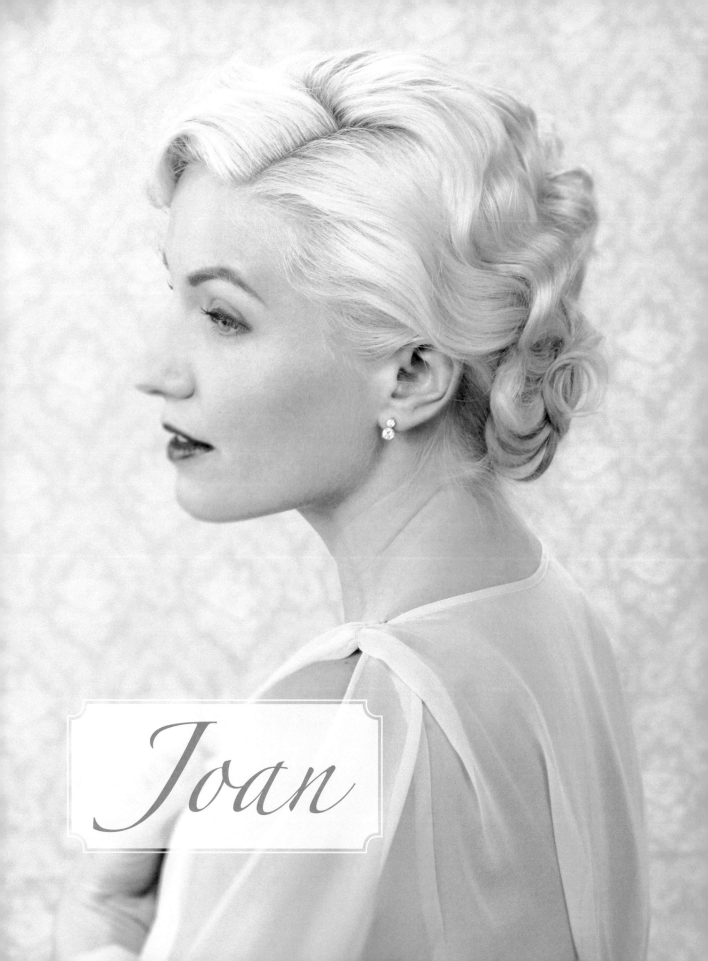

Joan

Supplies

thermal hair setting spray
hairspray
pomade
hair dryer
hair dryer diffuser
   attachment

¾" curling iron
¾ - ½" tapered curling iron
carbon tail comb
styling brush
loop and tail styling tool
grip bob pins

ripple hair pins
duckbill clips
hair clips
small rubber band
hair net with elastic
playing cards

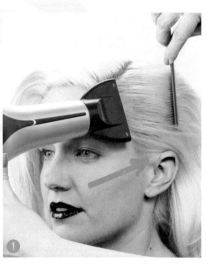
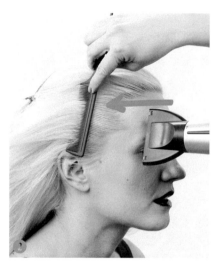

1 Prep the hair using the steps described on page 22 for setting product into the hair.

2 Use a comb and hair dryer to base direction blow-dry the hair around the front hairline back away from the face. This is important for the hair around the face to lay properly.

3 Part out these 5 sections. The front hairline is divided into 3 equal sections, about 2 inches deep and 3-4 inches wide. One is directly on top and runs from the part above the outer corner of the left eyebrow over to above the outer corner of the right eyebrow. The other 2 run from the first section down to the tops of the ears. The 4th section is a round section at the back of the crown. The 5th section is the rest of the hair at the back of the head.

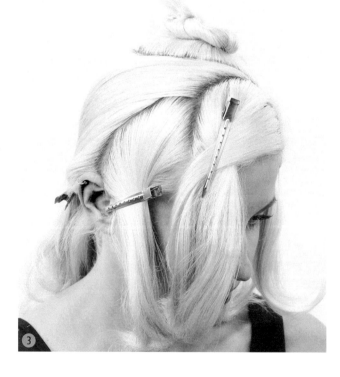

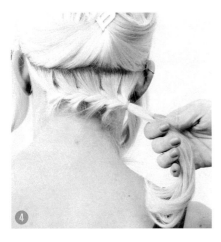
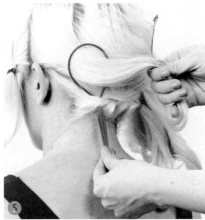
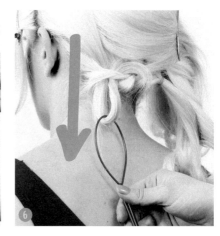

4 Braid a 1 inch thick horizontal section at the nape of the neck into a French braid and secure it with a small rubber band.

5 Using a loop and tail styling tool pull a thin, long piece of section 5 on the left back of the head through the braid.

6 Pull the ends all the way through.

7 Continue in small sections across the back of the head pulling small sections of hair through the braid.

8 Move to the left side of the head. Curl the section on the left side. This piece includes the hair to the left of the part down to the ear. Part out 3 long, thin pieces for curling.

Use the ¾ - ½" tapered curling iron in your right hand with the wand pointing straight down the floor. Curl using the left wrap pattern for a tapered curling iron as described on page 21. Use caution not to burn your fingers.

9 Clip the curls to cool.

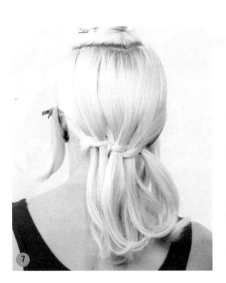
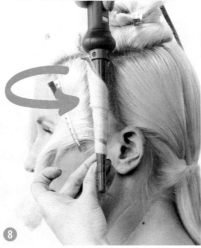
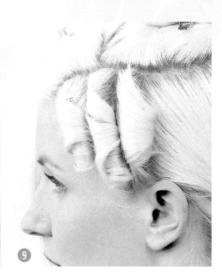

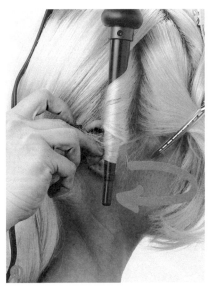

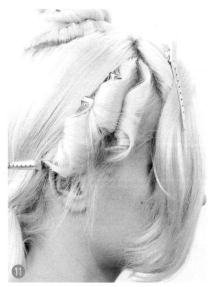

10 Move to the section on the right side. Holding the tapered curling iron in you left hand with the wand pointing straight down the floor, curl the hair using the right wrap pattern as described on page 20. Use caution not to burn your fingers.

11 Curl this section in 3 thin slices. Clip the curls to cool.

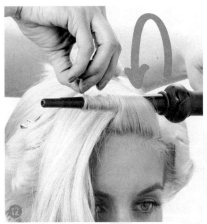

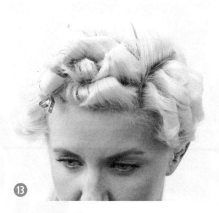

12 Next, curl the top section. With the tapered curling iron in your left hand holding it horizontal to the floor, curl using the right wrap pattern.

13 Clip the curls to cool.

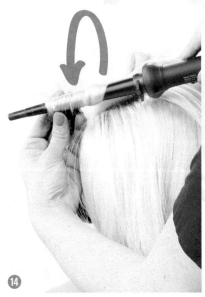

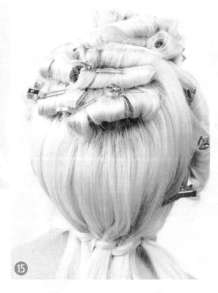

14 The last section left to work with is section 4 at the back of the crown. Holding the tapered curling iron in your right hand with the wand horizontal to the floor, curl using the left wrap pattern.

15 Clip the curls to cool.

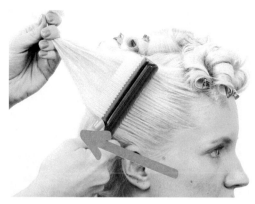

16 The waves of this hairstyle overlap each other, so it is important to brush out the section that will be on the bottom first and work you way to the top. Starting on the right, brush the section back to start spreading the wave.

17 After you have brushed, hang on the ends of the section and release some of the tension. You will start to see the wave take shape.

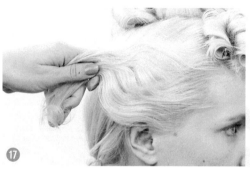

18 Back-comb the section to start spreading the wave and locking the hairs together.

19 Comb the hair against the head to start forming it into a wave. Comb up and down in a wave pattern to guide and manipulate the wave.

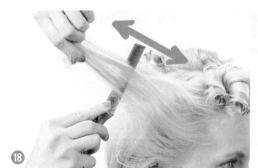

20 Clip the deepest parts of the waves with duckbill clips to enhance the shape. Use pieces of playing cards between the clips and the hair to avoid marks.

21 Heat the wave up with the hair dryer diffuser attachment and then allow it to cool to help set the wave.

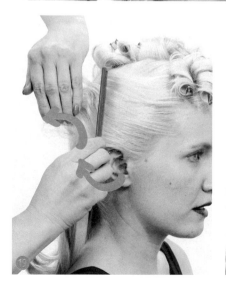

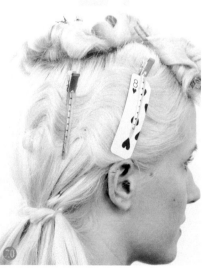

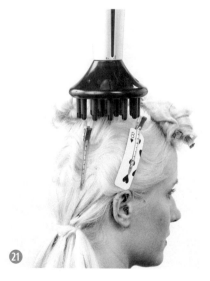

77

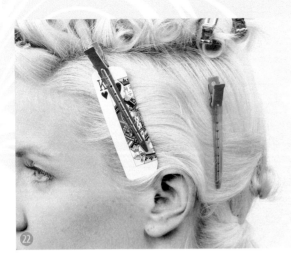

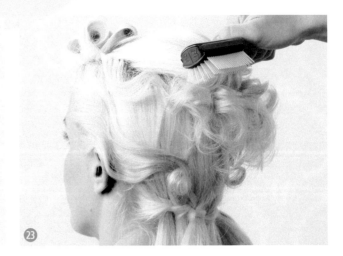

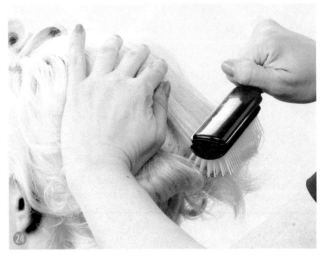

22 On the left side, repeat the steps 16-21 on the previous page. Brush the section back, back-comb to spread the wave and lock the hairs together. Comb the hair against the head to start forming it into a wave. Comb up and down in a wave pattern to guide the hair. Clip the deepest parts of the waves with duckbill clips to enhance the shape. Heat the wave up with the hair dryer diffuser attachment and then allow it to cool to help set the wave.

23 Next, brush out the section that was curled at the back of the crown.

24 Brush straight back. Try to avoid accidentally grabbing any of the hair underneath that has been looped through the lower braid. These waves are to sit on top of this section, not be brushed into it. Use your hands to help smooth the wave down and spread it around the back of the hairstyle.

25 You can clip the deepest parts of these waves with duckbill clips to enhance the shape or leave it for a softer look.

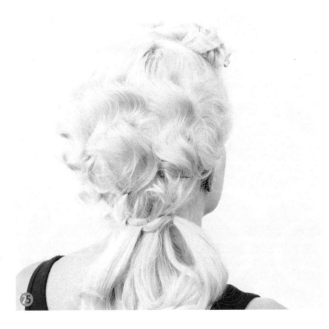

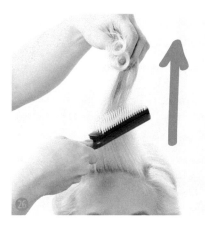
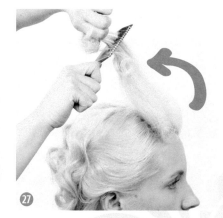
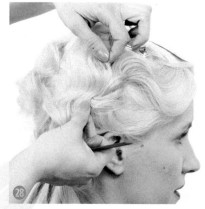

26   On the top section above the forehead, brush the section back and to the right.

27   Back-comb to spread the wave and lock the hairs together. Comb the hair against the head to start forming it into a wave. Comb left and right in a wave pattern to guide and manipulate. Arrange the wave to cascade some down the face.

28   Hide the ends of this piece by pulling them back to the back waves and overlapping these back waves over the ends. Use grip bob pins to secure.

29   The last step is to finish the back of the hairstyle. This lower back area is important in hiding the ends of the back wave that are still visible. Curl the hair looped through the lower braid with the ¾" curling iron.

30   Working in small sections, twist the ends of the hair hanging down up into the nape in a pin curl or floral pattern. Arrange the curls to cover any unsightly parts.

31   Use grip pins to secure. If the hair is too short here, use hair sewing to secure the style. See page 26 for more information on sewing hair.

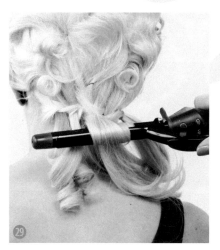
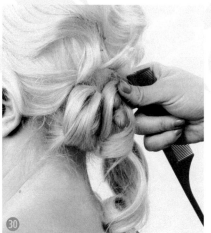
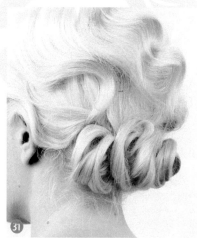

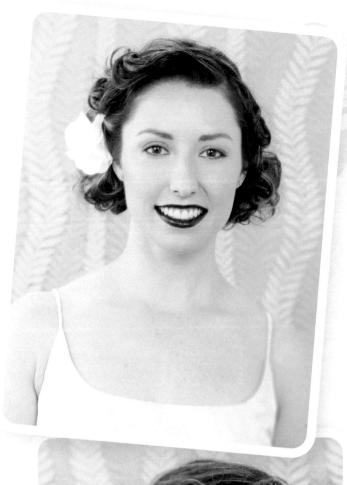

Lillian is a great hairstyle for a 1930s look on someone with lots of long hair. Although this model's hair is not very long, this hairstyle could easily be adapted.

In the 1930s, the bobbed waves close to the scalp silhouette gave way to a looser, fuller bob style. It is a nice, soft alternative and requires less precision in combing and arranging the hair.

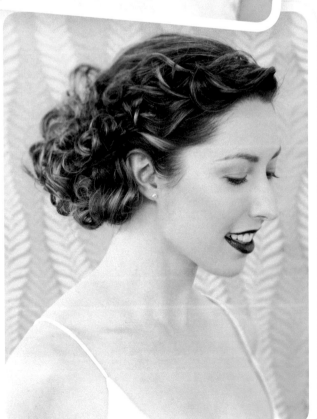

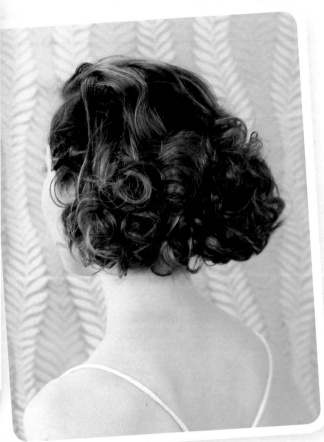

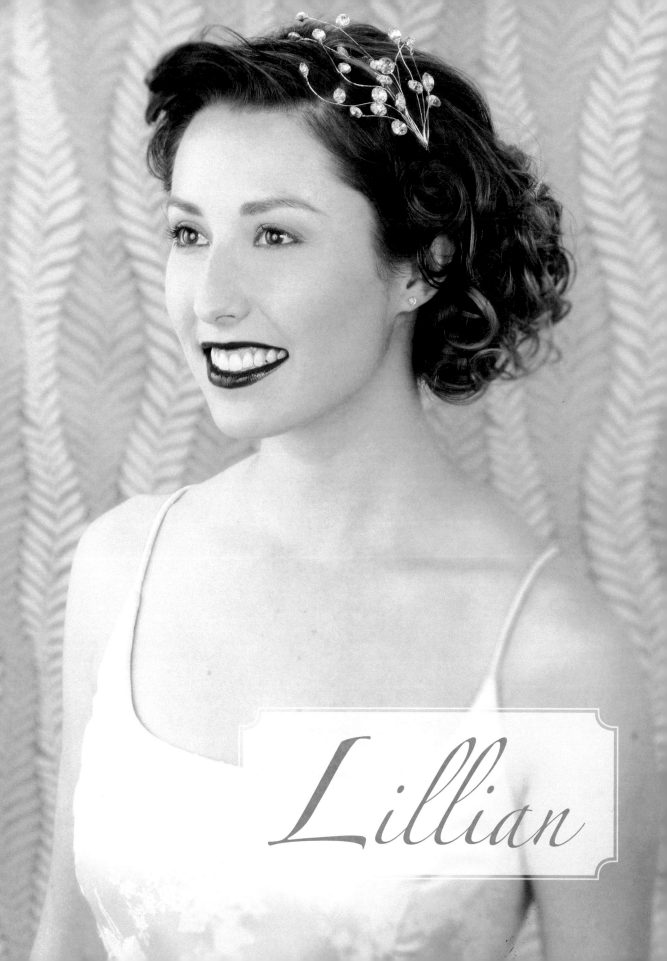

Lillian

Supplies

thermal hair setting spray
hairspray
pomade
hair dryer

hot sticks
carbon tail comb
wide tooth comb
grip bob pins

ripple hair pins
small rubber band
end wraps

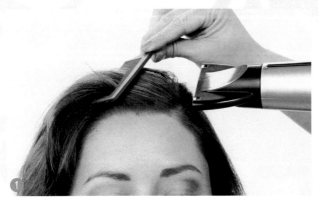

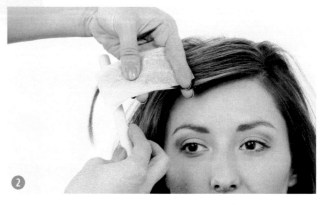

1 Prep the hair using the steps described on page 22 for setting product. Use the steps described on page 23 to set the part above the outer corner of the left eyebrow.

2 Direct the hair to the right for the first curl. End wraps help get stray ends around the very small circumference of a hot stick roller.

3 Set the first curl in a hot stick.

4 The next 2 curls come out of the section to the left of the part. When preparing each piece to curl, direct the hair back so that it lines up horizontally with the floor, hold the roller perpendicular to the floor and roll forward toward the face.

5 Set the rest of the hair in a horizontal bricklay pattern. When you reach the nape of the neck, leave a 2 inch deep section free.

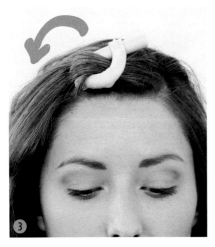

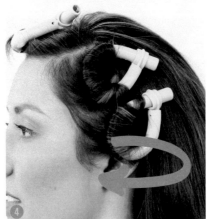

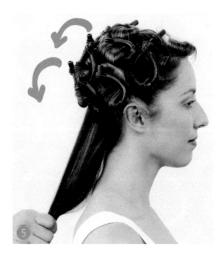

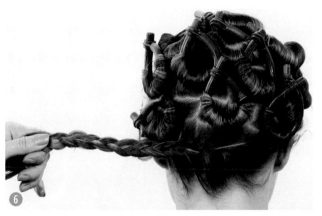

6 Braid the lower section across into a horizontal French braid and secure the end with a small rubber band.

7 Twist the end of the braid to overlap the scalp and use grip bob pins to secure it in a tight mass.

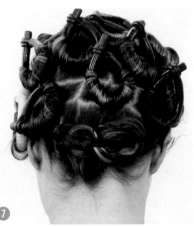
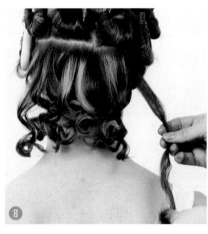
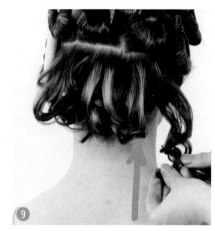

8 Begin removing the hot sticks a row at a time starting at the bottom. Using a small amount of pomade on your fingers, separate the curls and define them.

9 On the first lower row, a piece at a time, insert a grip bob pin to the end of the curls and pin them up underneath into the braid to start forming the faux bob.

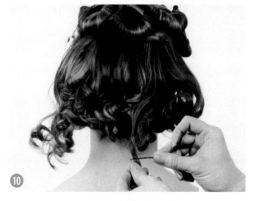

10 Let down the next row of hot stick curls. Separate the curls and define them with your fingers. Insert a grip bob pin to the end of the curls.

11 Pin the curls one at a time, this time a little higher above the nape, locking them into the layer just below it. The attempt is to create a mass of curl that slowly graduates up the back.

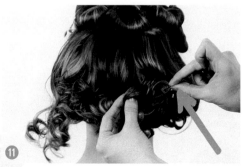

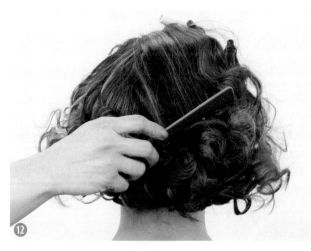

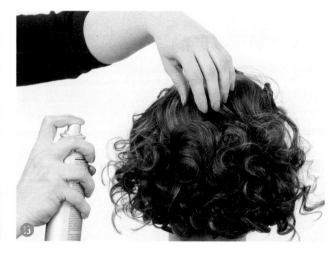

12 Release the last hot sticks on the back of the hairstyle. Comb gently with a wide tooth comb.

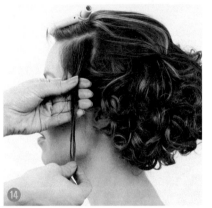

13 Arrange the curls with your fingers. Pin where needed to create balance and uniformity in the shape. The form and movement of the mass of curls in this hairstyle is focused in a sweep to the back.

14 Release the 2 curls set on the left side. Using a small amount of pomade on your fingers, separate the curls and define them.

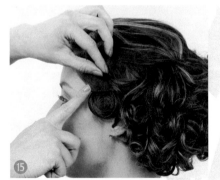

15 Direct the lower curl back above the ear to continue the sweeping back motion and grip pin to secure.

16 Arrange the higher curl into a pin curl that sits close to the scalp and grip pin to secure.

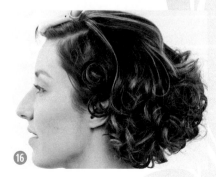

17 Release the last few curls on the right side of the hairstyle. Using a small amount of pomade on your fingers, separate the curls and define them. Using your fingers, grip the curls so the hair lays tightly against the scalp and direct the curls back to accumulate behind the ear. Grip pin to secure.

18 Remove the final roller at the top above the eyebrows. Separate the curls and direct them back and to the right.

19 Arrange this piece to sweep back and pin in place.

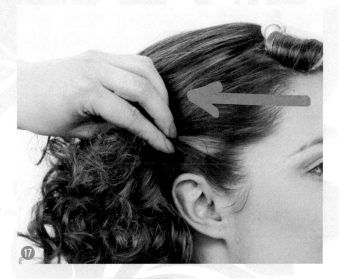

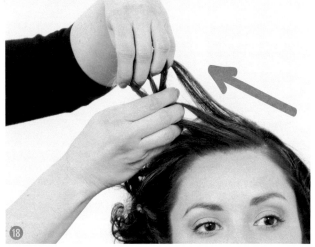

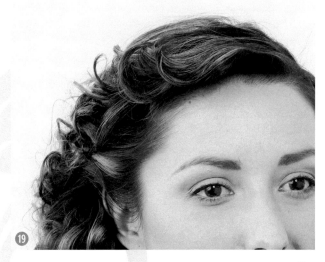

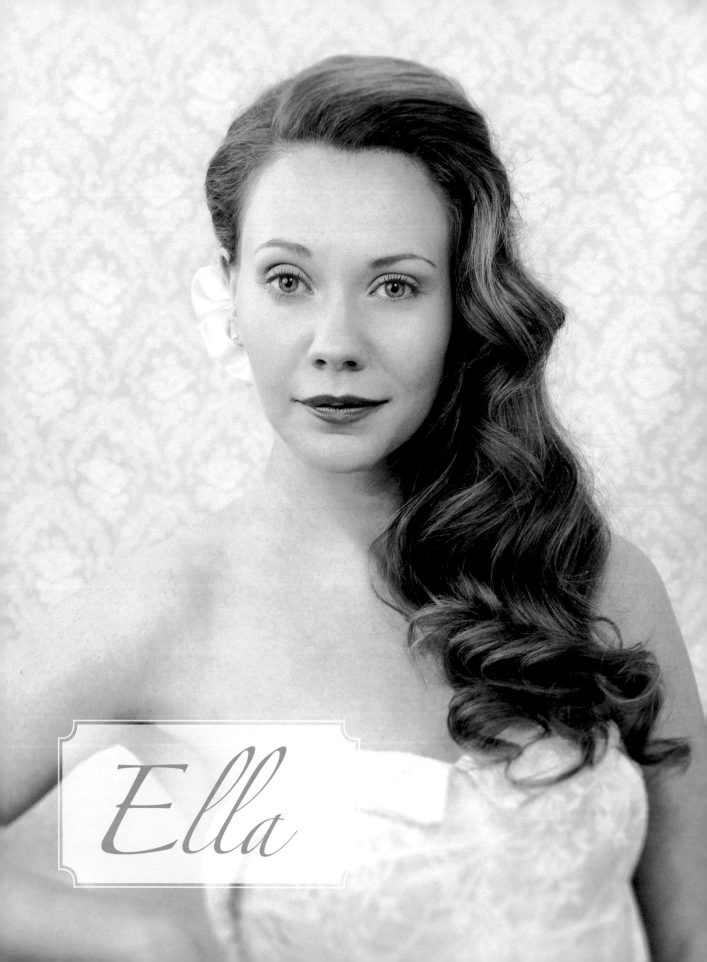

Ella

At a formal event, a loose down style can be problematic. As you move and dance and sweat, the curls can breakdown. What you saw in the mirror can quickly change into a flat mess. With the **Ella** slyle, pinning the hair in the back keeps it slightly contained. It gives the feel of a down hairstyle with the control of an up-do.

The Ella style design is a great option for someone with fine hair who wants the full, long waves of a 1940s hairstyle. Various sized curling irons will give you different waves on different hair textures, so test the curling iron before committing to the size.

The waves with curled ends in the Ella style are formed by wrapping the hair around the curling iron in a very specific way. Practice the steps with a cool curling iron before attempting on the hair to protect it. Since the delicate ends of the hair spend the most time on the hot curling iron, it is best to be comfortable and fast with the curl.

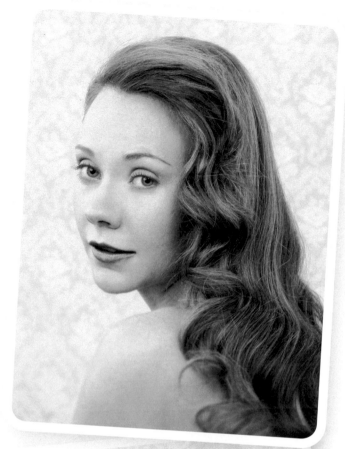

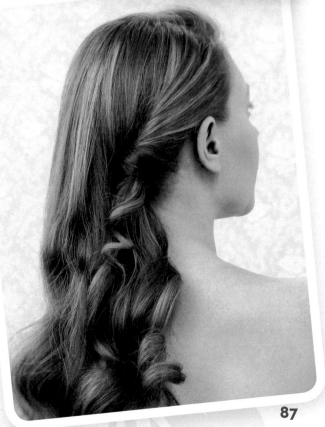

Supplies

volume spray
thermal hair setting spray
hairspray
pomade
hair dryer

¾" curling iron
carbon tail comb
round vent brush
styling brush

grip bob pins
ripple hair pins
duckbill clips
hair clips

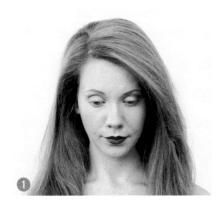

1. Prep the hair using the steps described on page 22. The Ella hairstyle should have some volume. Try to eliminate any unruly growth patterns at the front hairline. Part above the right eyebrow. Do not base direction blow-dry the part.

2. To set the front of the hairstyle, separate a section 1 inch deep that runs from the part on the right over the left side of the head to above the left eyebrow. Part this section out into long, diagonal parts for curling.

Using a ¾" curling iron, curl the hair using these important steps. This is not a traditional curling iron curl. It is similar to the tapered wand wrap on page 20, but with 2 key differences. The curl begins at the end of the hair and the curling iron will move around the hair as opposed to the hair moving around the curling iron.

Practice this curl with a cool curling iron before attempting on the hair to protect it. Since the delicate ends of the hair spend the most time on the hot curling iron, it is best to be comfortable and fast with the curl before it counts.

3. Hold the first piece of hair between your left fingers. Hold the iron in your right with the wand pointing up and the shell facing the rear. Clamp the shell around the end.

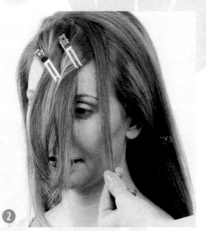
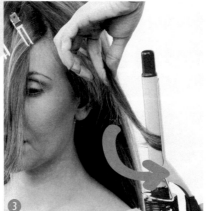
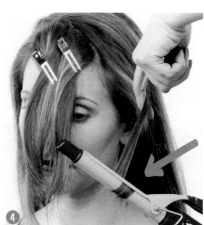

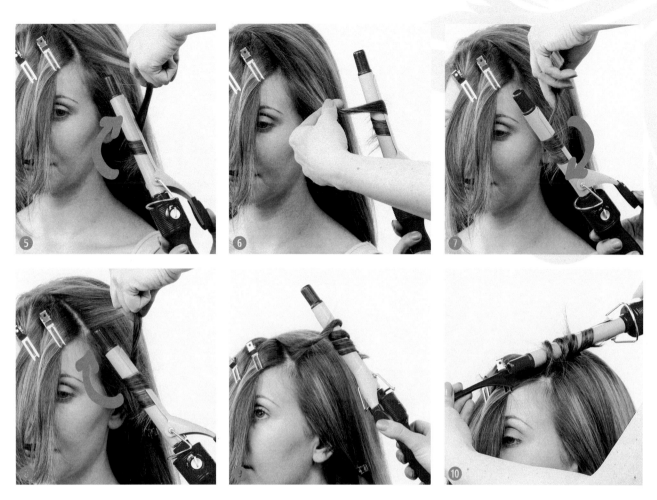

4 Hold the hair strands stationary with your left hand and begin to twirl the curling iron around the hair strands to the left.

5 Spin the curling iron under to the right so it passes between the hair strand and the scalp.

6 The curling iron has made one full rotation around the piece of hair.

7 Continue to twirl the curling iron around to the left for another rotation around the hair strands.

8 Spin the curling iron under to the right so it passes between the hair strand and the scalp.

9 Keep twirling and you will notice the hair is twisting as it circles the curling iron.

10 For these top 3 curls, it is important to curl as much of the strand as possible. Keep attempting the twirl until it is no longer possible. If there is still some uncurled hair at the base, protect the scalp with a comb between it at the iron and rotate the curling iron up to curl the last of the base. Clip the curl to cool.

11 Begin the next curl the same as described in step 3.

12 Follow steps 4-10 to twist the curl around the curling iron. Clip the curl to cool.

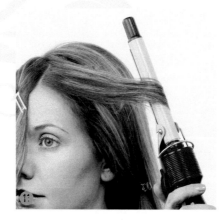 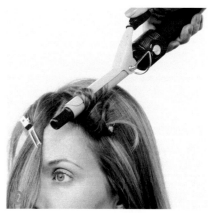

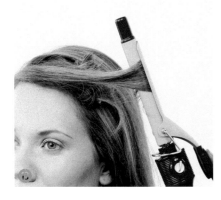 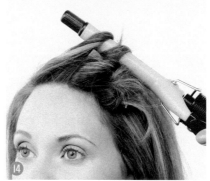 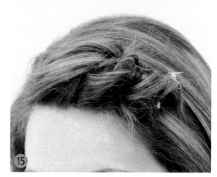

13 Begin the final curl next to the part the same way as described in step 3.

14 Follow steps 4-10 to twist the curl around the curling iron. Clip the curl to cool.

15 There are 3 identical curls in the fringe area.

16 The rest of the hairstyle will be curled with this twist curl going the opposite direction. The first curl starts with a long, thin sliced section that reaches from the bottom of the curls just set down to the ear.

17 Hold this first piece of hair between your left fingers. Hold the iron in your

right with the wand pointing up and the shell facing forward. Clamp the shell around the end.

18 Similar to the first curls, hold the hair strands stationary with your left hand, but twirl the curling iron around the hair strands to the right.

19 Direct the curling iron under and to the left so that it passes between the hair strand and the scalp.

20 Continue to twirl the curling iron around to the right.

21 Twirl the curling iron under and to the left so that it passes between the hair strand and the scalp.

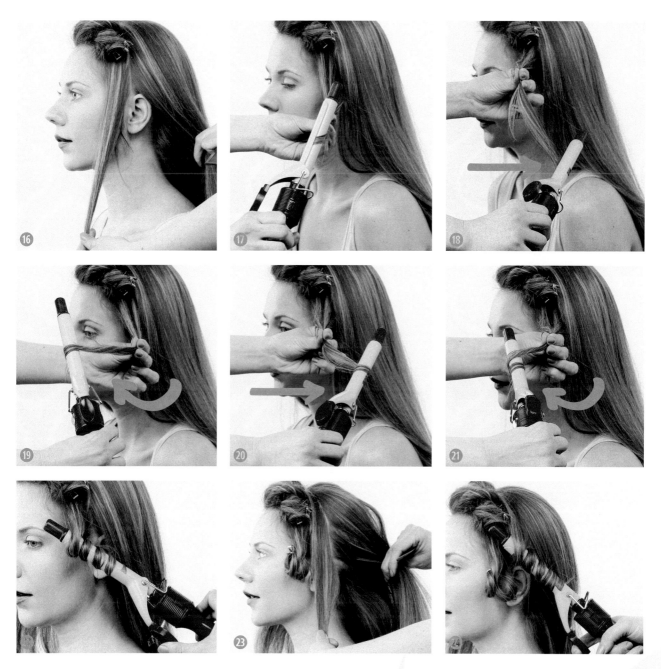

22   These curls will end slightly different. Before, the goal was to the curl all the way to the scalp. Here, these curls which will rotate around the rest of the hairstyle, will stop at a point that aligns with the lower hairline. When the curling iron reach the height of the hairline below the curl, finish, release the curl, and clip it to cool.

23   Take the next long, thin section that begins at the part on the top of the head.

24   Follow steps 17-22 to curl the section.

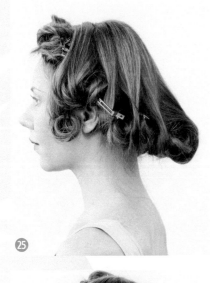

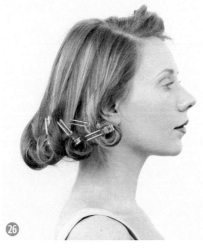

25 Continue to take long, thin sections of hair that spray out from the part at the top of the head and curl them using the steps 17-22.

26 Continue until you reaching the right side of the head. The curls should all end at the hairline and so the clipped curls will all sit at the lower hairline.

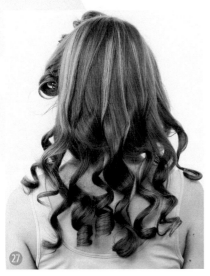

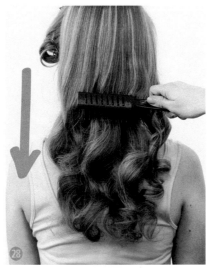

27 Remove the hair clips from the lower level of curls.

28 Brush them out gently with a styling brush.

29 Brush straight down to the floor to define the wave.

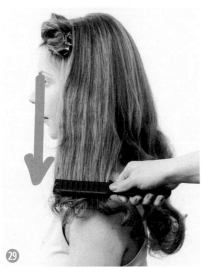

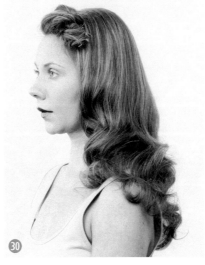

30 Because the curls were all created in line with each other and in the same direction, the wave will be uniform.

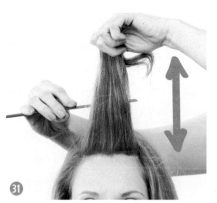
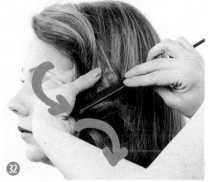
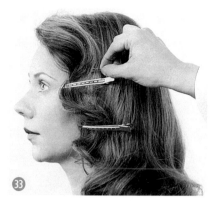

31 Remove the hair clips from the curls above the forehead. Comb the curls in one mass straight up from the scalp.

32 Bring the section over to the left side of the head and comb and arrange the wave.

33 Clip the deepest parts of the waves with duckbill clips to enhance the shape. Use grip pins to secure the wave in position.

34 On the right side of the hairstyle, separate out a section from the part on the right down to the nape of the neck. Twist it up away from the neck and grip pin it in place to secure it.

35 Back-comb the hair on the left.

36 Fold the hair to the right close to the twist and grip pin it in place.

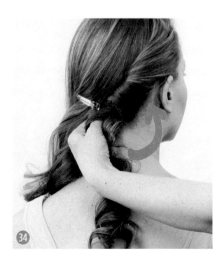
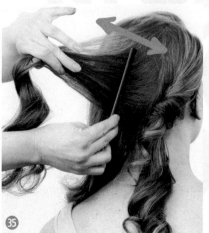
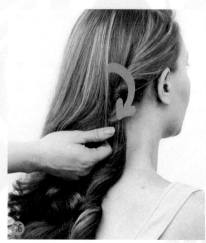

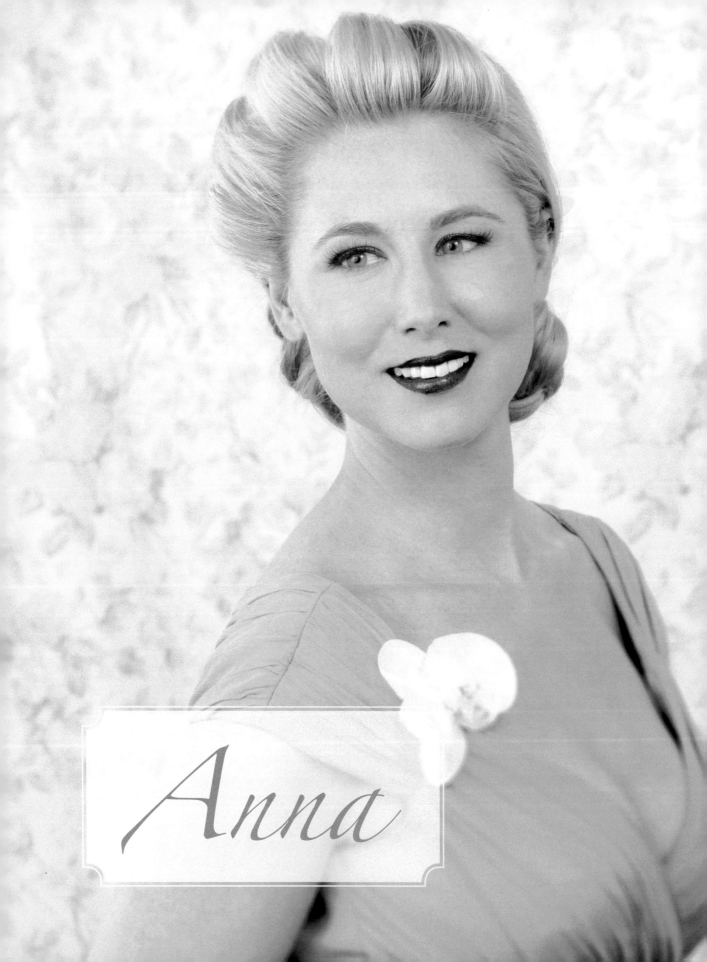

Anna

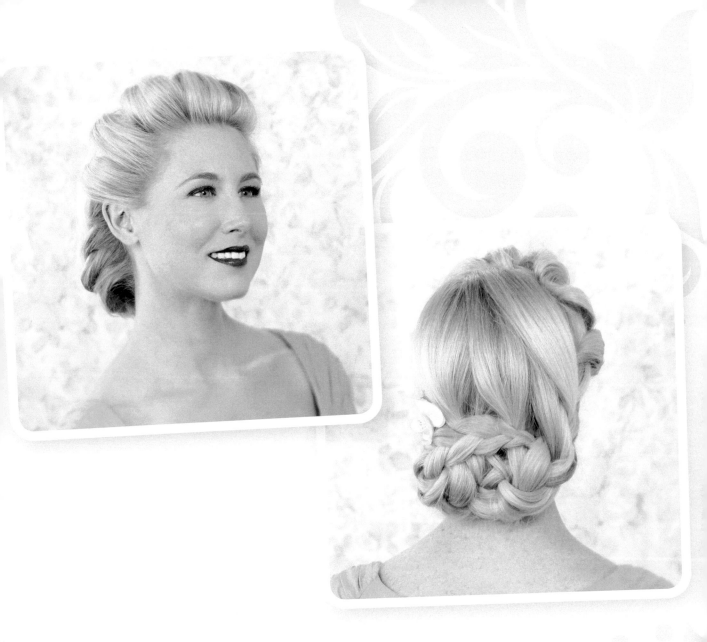

When you are low on time and someone with lots of thick hair needs a fast hairstyle, the **Anna** hairstyle can be a lifesaver. It needs no curling iron and it contains a lot of hair quickly with beautiful texture.

The 1940s silhouette is based on a regulation hairstyle for a woman during WWII. It was a common silhouette for women who needed to keep their hair above the collar and out of the way for war work. It also frames the face beautifully for photographs.

Supplies

volume spray	hair dryer	grip bob pins
thermal hair setting spray	carbon tail comb	ripple hair pins
hairspray	round vent brush	duckbill clips
pomade	styling brush	small rubber band

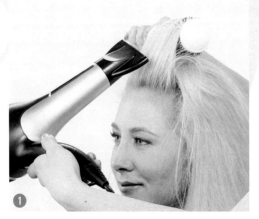

1 Prep using the steps described on page 22 for setting product into the hair. Use a volume blow-dry to eliminate any unruly growth patterns and add volume to the front hairline. Part above the left eyebrow.

2 Take a section from the part 2 inches deep from above the left eyebrow down to the right ear Create 5 small, equal sections from this larger section and clip them for future styling.

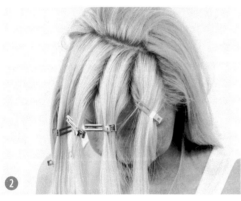

3 Take the first 2 pieces in your right and left hand and hold them up straight from the scalp.

4 Cross them over each other loosely 2 times.

5 Bend the twist back behind itself and use a grip bob pin to secure it to the hair at the scalp. Be sure to preserve the volume at the front hairline. Let the ends hang down to the right side behind everything.

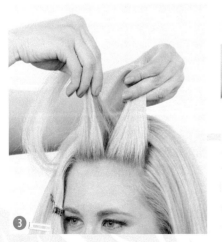
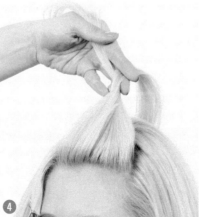
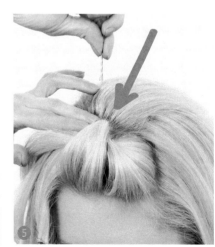

6 Repeat these steps on the next 2 pieces. Take the pieces in your right and left hand and hold them straight out and slightly up from the scalp. Cross them over each other loosely 2 times.

7 Bend the twist back behind the two sections and the ends hanging down from the previous section. Use a grip bob pin to secure the twist to the hair at the scalp. Be sure to preserve the volume at the front hairline.

8 Hold the last piece that is directly above the right ear straight out from the scalp.

9 Arch the piece back behind itself and the ends hanging down from the previous sections. Preserve the volume so that when you look at the front of the finished style, there appears to be a crown of hair spraying out from the forehead.

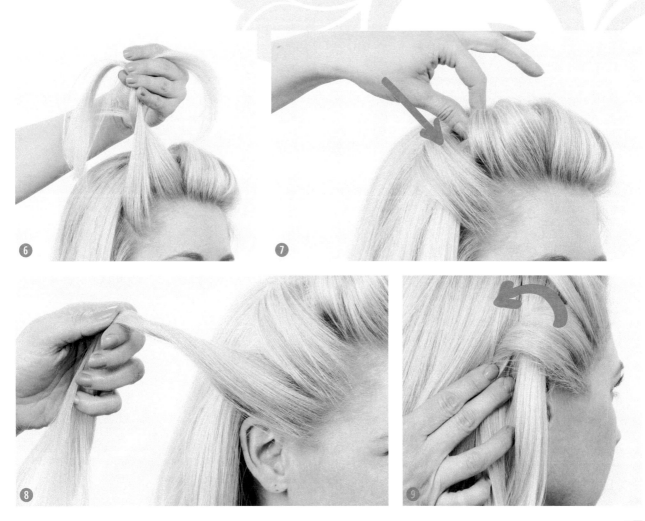

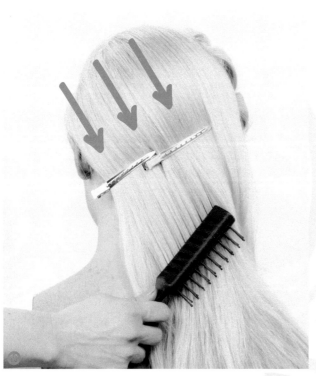

10 Brush all of the rest of the hair, including the unused hair above the left ear tightly over in a diagonal to the right. It helps the get the teeth of the brush well down into the hair at the scalp. All of this hair will be used in the next step. Use duckbill clips to keep the hair in position and ready for use.

11 Start a French braid behind the right ear using slices of hair that radiate from the part above the left eyebrow and include the ends of the hair from the twists created on the previous page.

12 Continue the French braid around along the hairline.

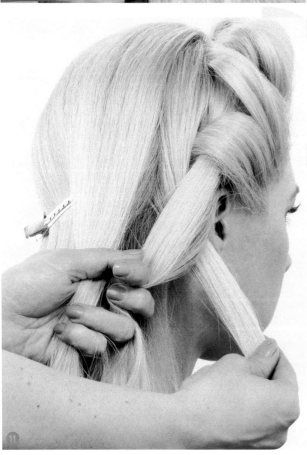

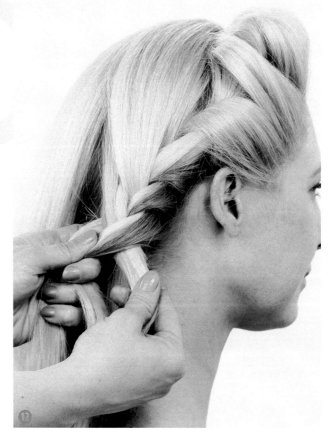

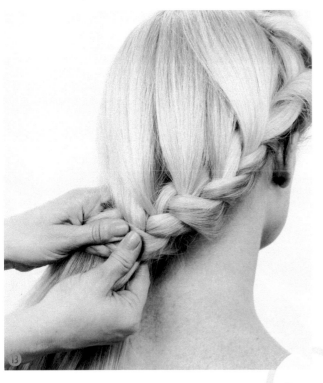

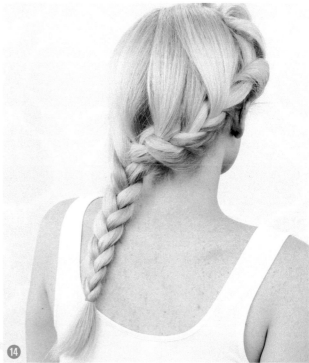

13 Continue to French braid along the hairline keeping the braid tight to the scalp. Form the slices of hair for your French braid using hair all the way from the part and left side of the head so that all of the hair makes it into the French braid.

14 Once you have reached the left side of the nape of the neck you should be finished with pulling the hair in from the front left side. There should be no lose hair left. Here, finish the braid down the back and secure with a small rubber band.

15 Curl the braid up to the nape and arrange it into its shape. Hide the end underneath and place grip bob pins through the braid to secure it.

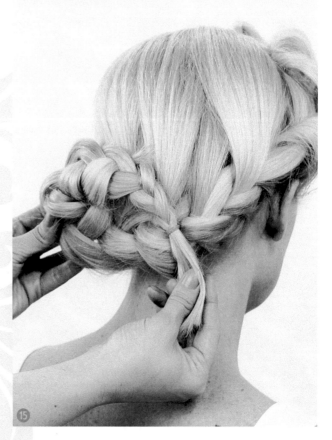

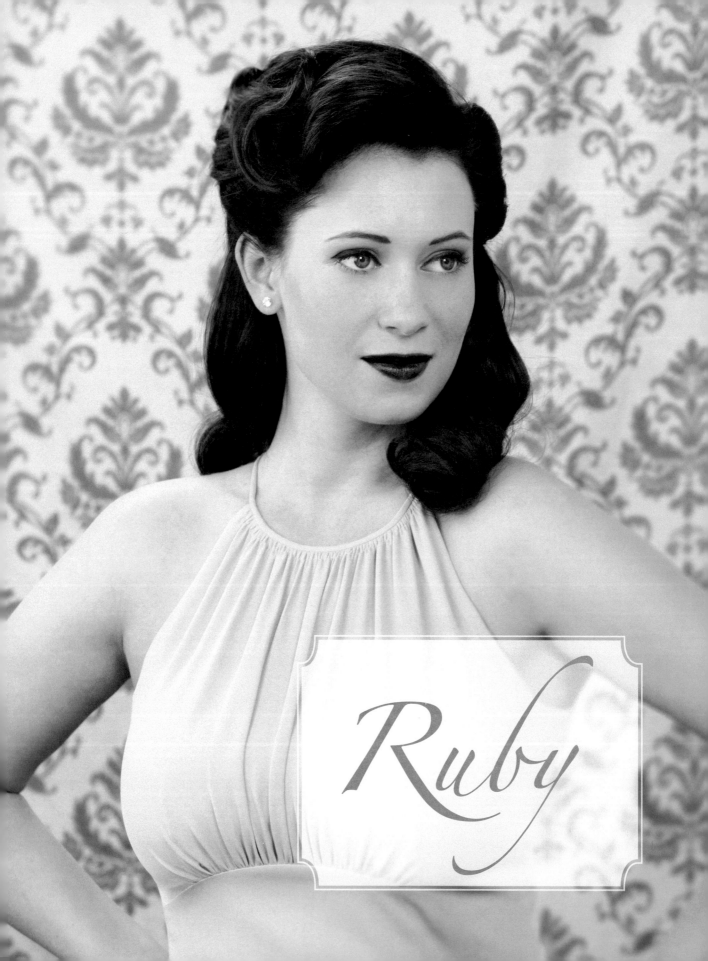

Ruby

The silhouette of the **Ruby** is a very popular one for girls looking for a 1940s style. The ease of it makes it a great hairstyle for a morning or afternoon wedding.

The sides are pinned up and the back falls down in a cascade of soft waves. These falling waves can be made into tighter curls to suit taste.

The undulating waves over the top of the crown provide a nice opportunity to mix things up as well. If you have a number of bridesmaids you would like to have similar looks without matching perfectly, this is a good option to play with.

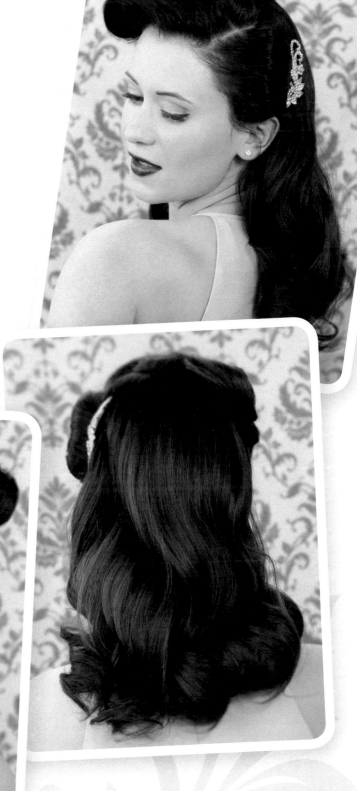

Supplies

volume spray
thermal hair setting spray
hairspray
pomade
1" curling iron

1 ¼" curling iron
carbon tail comb
wide tooth comb
styling brush
grip bob pins

ripple hair pins
duckbill clips
hair clips
hair filler

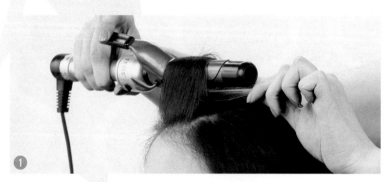

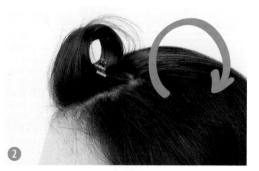

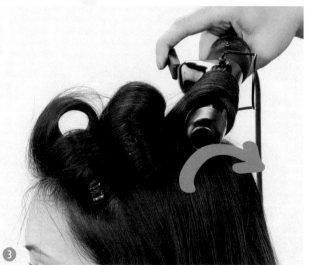

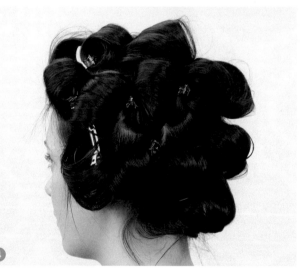

1 Prep using the steps described on page 22 for setting product into the hair. Use a volume blow-dry to eliminate any unruly growth patterns and add volume to the front hairline. Part above the left eyebrow. Use a 1" curling iron to curl on-base curls for the first few curls on top. They should be a tighter curl.

2 Clip the curls to cool.

3 Switch to 1 ¼" curling iron once you reach the back of the crown.

4 Curl the rest of the hair with larger 1 ¼" curling iron. Remove the clips once the curls have cooled.

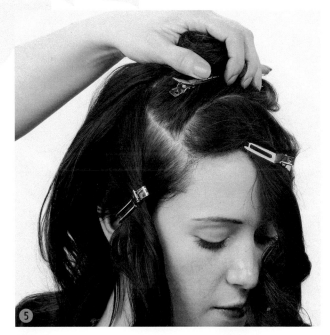

5 Separate the hair into 5 sections as follows: a section above each ear that is about 3 inches tall by 2 inches deep and 2 rectangular sections above the forehead about 1 inch deep that stretch from above each eyebrow. The final section is the entire back of the head.

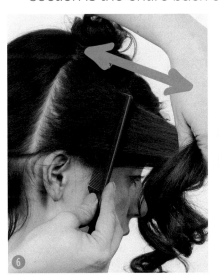

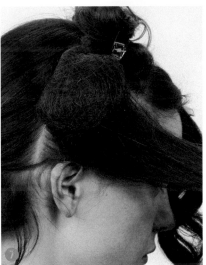

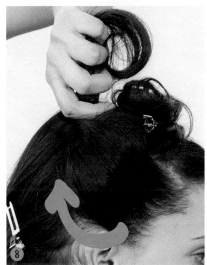

6 Begin with the right side section. Comb it forward toward the face and back-comb at the scalp to provide an anchor for grip pins.

7 Grip pin a thin, oblong hair filler over the hair at the scalp above the ear. See page 24 for more about creating a hair filler. The hair filler here is used for the illusion of some volume on the sides. It also provides a place to anchor hairpins for a longer lasting style.

8 Wrap the hair back around behind the hair filler to cover it and grip pin anchoring into the filler.

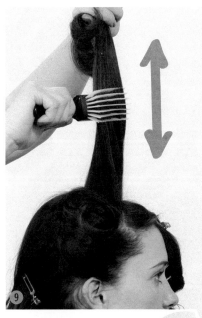

9 Work next with the section on top that is further toward the back. Brush the entire section out straight up from the scalp. Back brush the section to start spreading the wave and locking the hairs together. Use a comb to smooth out the hairs on the visible part of the section.

10 Bend it loosely down to the right and arrange it in a large wave and secure the curl configuration covering any visible parts to the rear of the hairstyle.

11 Anchor grip pins into the wave to secure it to the scalp hair below.

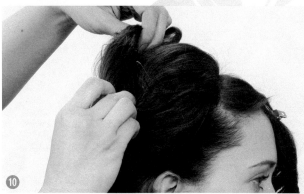

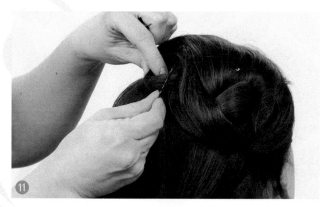

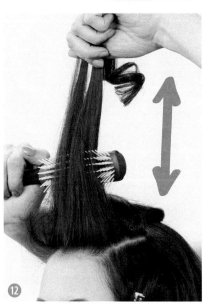

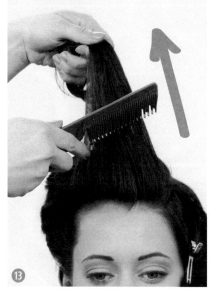

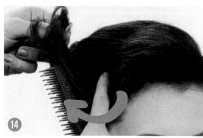

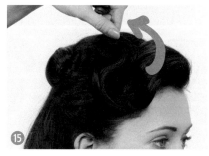

12 Repeat these steps on the forward section above the forehead. Brush the entire section out straight up from the scalp. Back brush the section to start spreading the wave and locking the hairs together.

13 Use a comb to smooth out the hairs on the visible part of the section.

14 Bend it loosely down to the right and arrange it in a large wave and secure the curl configuration.

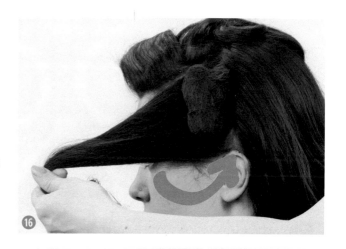

15 Manipulate the hair into the desired shapes and waves. Use ripple pins to hold the form while you work with it. Once you have the desired shape, insert grip pins in place of the ripple pins. See page 28 for more information about using ripple pins.

16 Comb the left section forward toward the face and back-comb at the scalp to provide an anchor for grip pins. Pin a thin, oblong hair filler over the hair at the scalp above the ear the same as you did in steps 6-7.

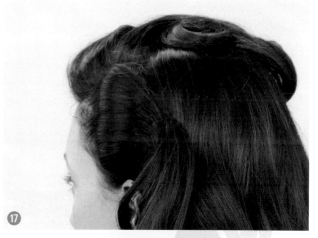

17 Wrap the hair back around behind the hair filler to cover it and grip pin anchoring into the filler.

18 Use a hair pick to gently comb out the last of the curls in the back. If there is still some time before the event, use a hair net or snood to encase the curls and keep them off the neck until later.

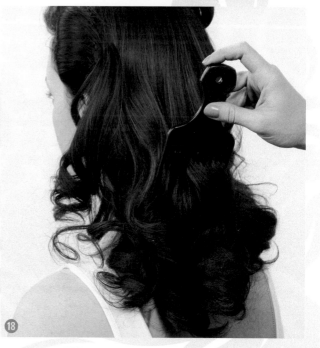

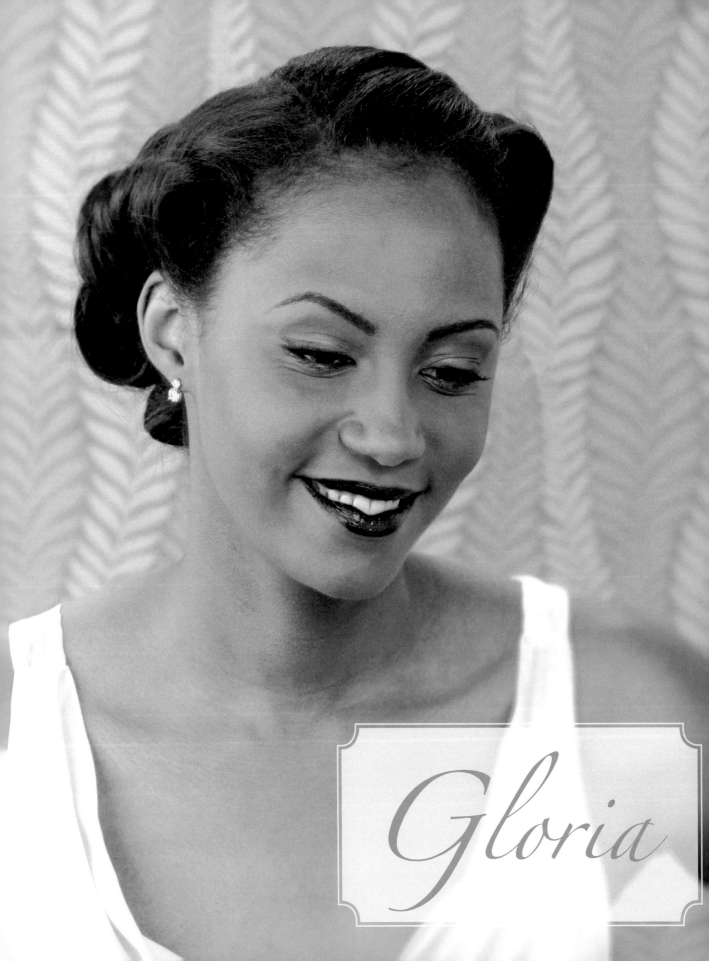

Gloria

The **Gloria** hairstyle plays on two iconic elements many people think of when they think of hair design of the 1940s: the victory roll and the continuous roll.

In this design, the victory rolls' diameter is a little smaller to keep balance between their size and the size of the rolls at the back of the style. They are also placed asymmetric in height to add some drama and variation for photographs.

A continuous roll is defined as one roll that stretches around the entire head, but the rolls of this style do not connect. Because the victory rolls curve back and disappear behind the ear, the style creates an illusion that they continue around the back.

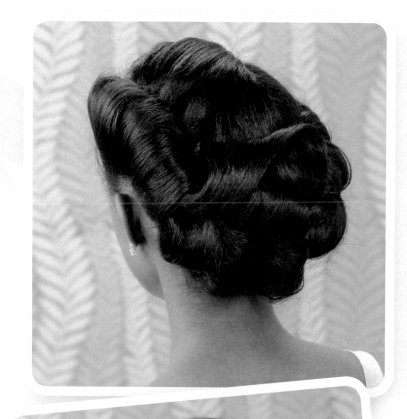

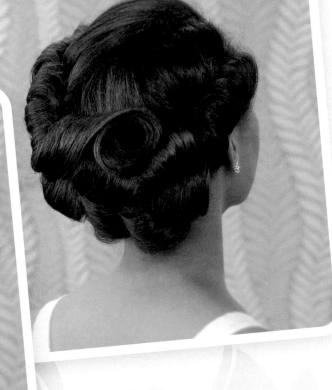

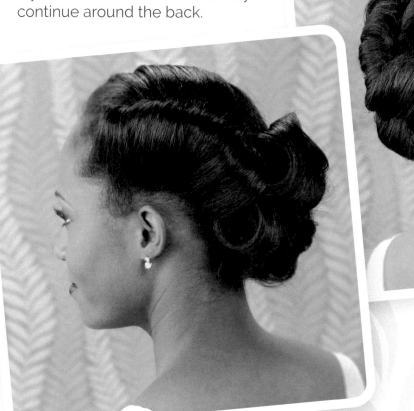

Supplies

thermal hair setting spray   hot rollers   grip bob pins
hairspray   carbon tail comb   ripple hair pins
pomade   loop and tail styling tool   small rubber bands
hair dryer

1 Prep using the steps described on page 22 for setting product into the hair. Using the steps described on page 23, use a base directional blow-dry around the lower level of the hairline up toward the crown.

2 With the base direction blow-dry, the victory rolls will not droop from gravity.

3 Blow-dry both sides above the ear upward.

4 Set the entire head in small hot rollers. Around the hairline just above the ears, roll the hot rollers up toward the crown.

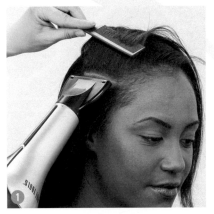
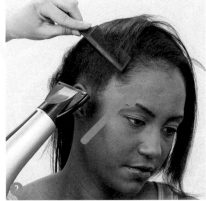
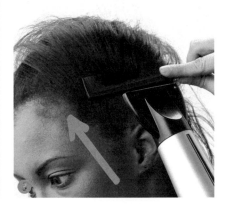
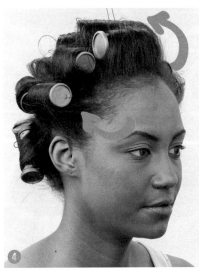
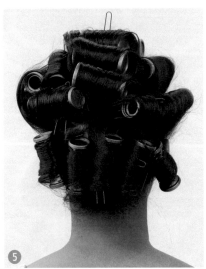
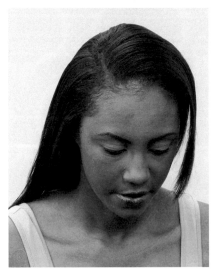

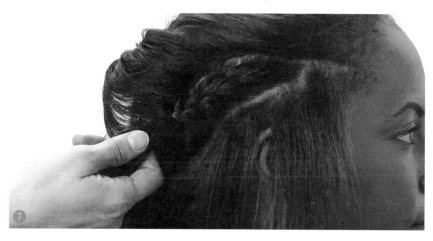

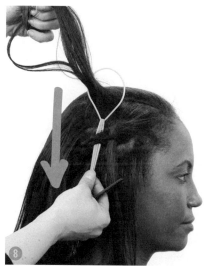

5 When setting the hot rollers at the crown, line them up and roll them back down to the occipital bone. Below the occipital bone, set the rollers perpendicular to the floor and roll them in toward the middle of the neck.

6 After the rollers have cooled, remove them. Part the hair above the outer corner of the right eye.

7 Create a diagonal arched scalp braid that will be hidden. To hide it, you will leave a 1 inch perimeter of hair around it free. Separate the section out beginning 1 inch below the part and 1 inch back from the front hairline. You will also leave a 1 inch area free below the braid. Braid back about 4 inches and then secure it at the base with a small rubber band.

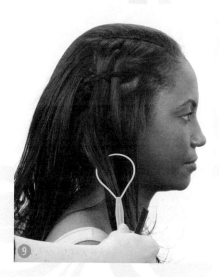

8 Using a loop and tail styling tool pull a thin, long section of the free hair above the braid down through it. Begin at the front hairline.

9 Pull the ends all the way through.

10 Continue with small sections, working back along the braid. Stop at the end of the braid.

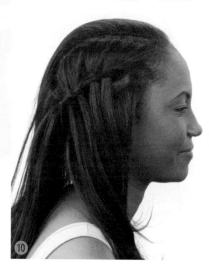

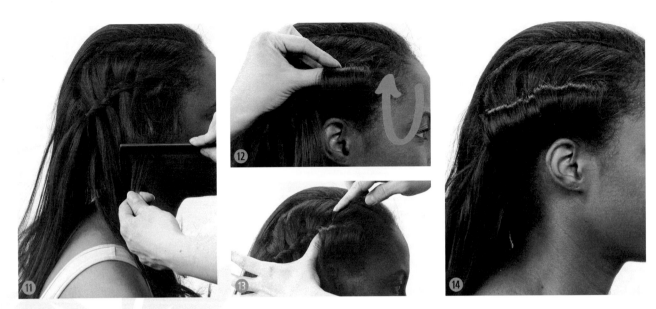

11 Back-comb the hair that is hanging down through and below the braid locking the hairs together. Smooth the side underneath that will be visible with the comb.

12 The victory roll will be created in small sections. With the hair pointing straight down toward the shoulder, start with about a 2 inch wide piece. Roll up beginning with the ends. The motion is similar to rolling an imaginary hot roller into the hair.

13 Secure it to the braid underneath with grip bob pins.

14 Continue with 1 inch sections rolling up until the braid is completely covered.

15 These same steps are used on the left side, but the perimeter around the braid is a little different. The braid still sits back 1 inch from the front hairline, but because the victory roll on the left will sit higher than the right, the braid needs to be higher. Leave about 2-3 inches of perimeter free below the braid. Braid in a diagonal arch .

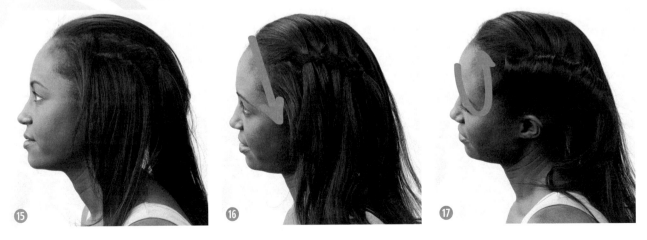

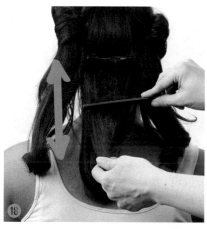
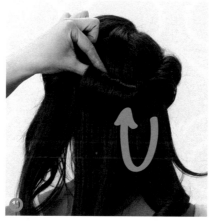
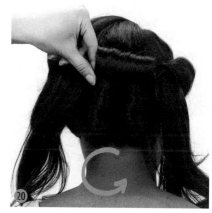

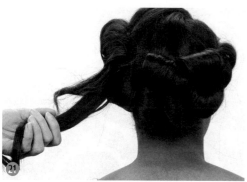

16 Repeat steps 8-10, pulling hair from the part above the right eye down through the braid using the loop and tail styling tool until you reach the end of the braid.

17 Repeat steps 11-14 to roll this hair into a long, continuous victory roll. If you follow the diagonal, the roll should appear to be arched.

18 Move to the back. Back-comb the hair that is hanging down locking the hairs together.

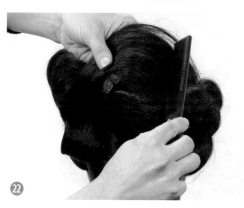

19 With about a 2 inch size piece, roll beginning with the ends toward the scalp, imagining that you are rolling a hot roller. Secure with grip bob pins at the base.

20 Set the hair at the nape in rolls perpendicular to the floor.

21 Continue setting everything in random victory rolls below the back of the crown, careful that they are arranged in a balanced way.

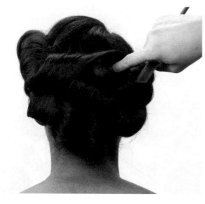

22 Not every piece of this hairstyle needs to be rolled into a victory roll.

23 To add some softness, a final piece at the occipital bone is styled in a wave ending in a pin curl.

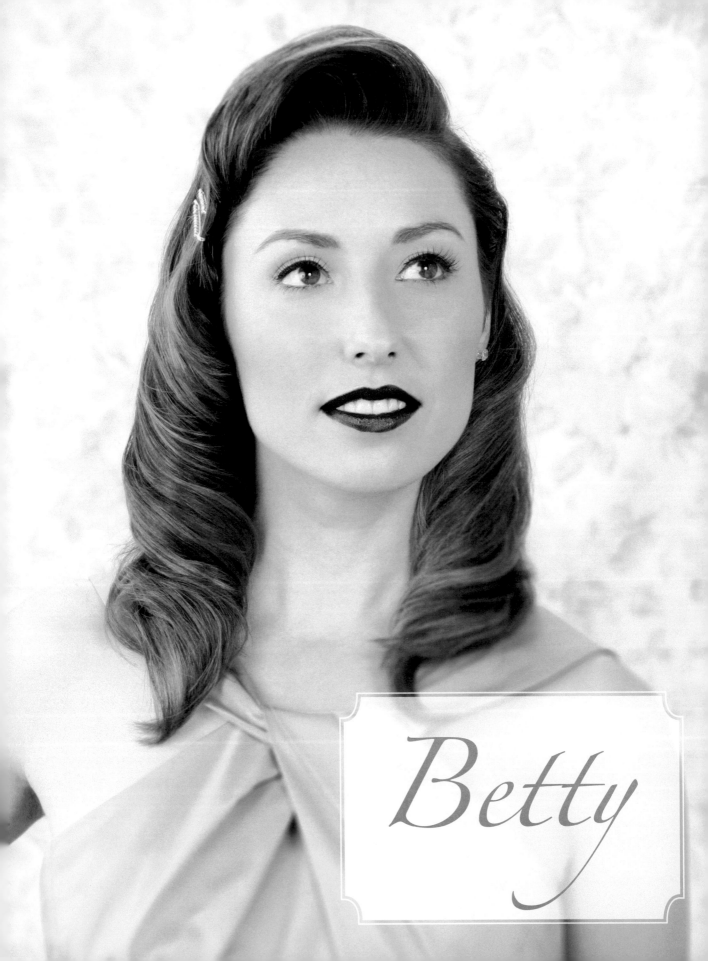

Betty

The **Betty** hairstyle, inspired by a 1940s pageboy, is great for any event. It is soft enough for a day wedding or garden party with a colorful dress, but also polished enough to look amazing with a biased-cut ivory wedding gown.

The preparation and base direction blow-dry for this style are important to keep it lying properly for an extended amount of time. If prepared properly, it will still look amazing a second day around.

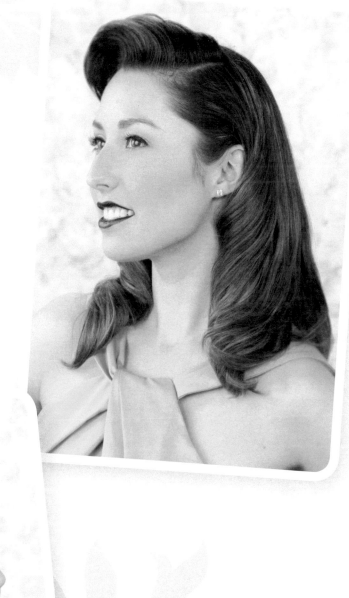

Supplies

volume spray
thermal hair setting spray
hairspray
pomade

hair dryer
flat iron
carbon tail comb
wide tooth comb

round vent brush
styling brush
grip bob pins
hair clips

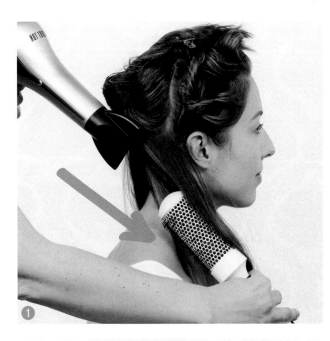

1 The blow-dry for the Betty is an important element to the hairstyle falling properly around the face. Prep using the steps described on page 22 for setting product into the hair, but follow the proceeding pattern for the base direction blow-dry.

Separate the hair into 4 sections; the back, the 2 sides above the ears, and the crown. Start the blow-dry at the lowest point and work your way up. Begin with the hair to the right side of the neck. Pointing the hair dryer nozzle at the nape of the neck, direct the hair forward around the neck toward the chin.

2 Then round brush blow-dry the section directing it forward.

With the section on the left side of the neck, use the same treatment except wrapping the hair around the left side of the neck and forward.

Continue this up the back of the head until you reach the crown.

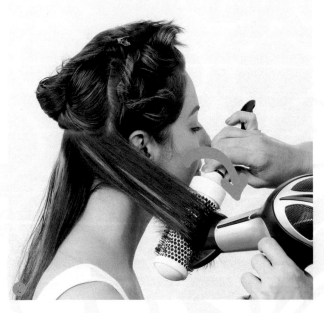

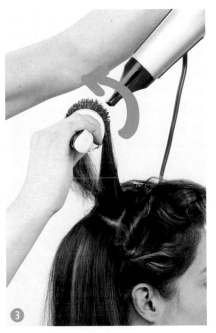

3 At the back of the crown, volume blow-dry the hair back.

4 On the right side above the ear, blow-dry in sections perpendicular to the floor. Direct the hair straight back, rolling the brush to the right so that the hair is swooping around the brush toward the chin. At the same time, blow-dry the hair at the scalp to direct straight back.

5 If done properly, the hair will make a c-shape around the ear. Repeat these steps to produce a reverse c-shape around the left ear.

6 On the last section at the top of the crown. Volume blow-dry the hair over the right.

7 Try to eliminate any unruly growth patterns at the front hairline above the forehead and direct the hair up and to the right while blow-drying.

8 The shape of the final style is partially visible after this blow-dry treatment.

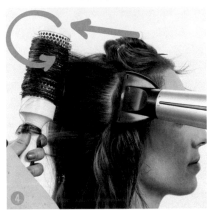

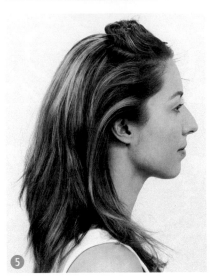

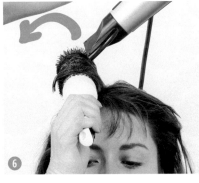

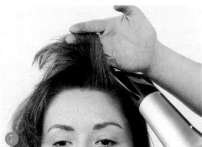

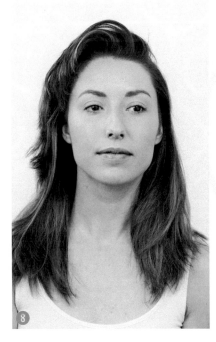

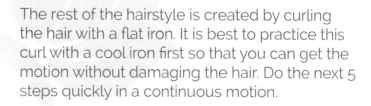

The rest of the hairstyle is created by curling the hair with a flat iron. It is best to practice this curl with a cool iron first so that you can get the motion without damaging the hair. Do the next 5 steps quickly in a continuous motion.

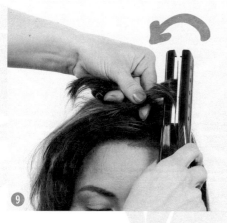

9 Starting with a section of hair above the forehead, clamp the flat iron down on the base of the hair.

10 Rotate the flat iron running it along the hair shaft in the direction you want the curl to rotate. This first curl rotates to the right. The flat iron does not get any further away from the scalp during this process. Similar to a curling iron curl, the hair is wrapping around the exterior of the flat iron.

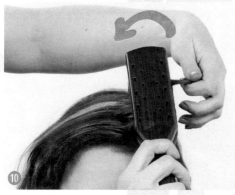

11 Continue to run the flat iron down the hair shaft while simultaneously rotating it in the direction of the curl.

12 When you have reached near the end, grab hold of the base to keep the curl from falling.

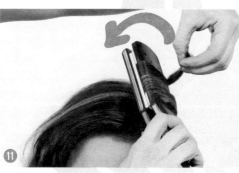

13 Use your hands to form the piece into a stand-up pin curl while it is still warm and clip the hair to cool in this shape.

14 Continue using this flat-iron curl on the hair above the forehead rotating the curls to the right.

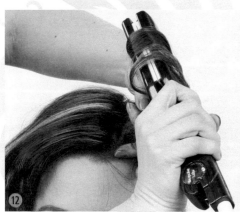
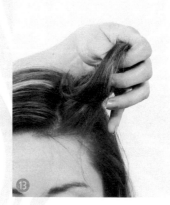
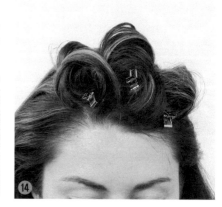

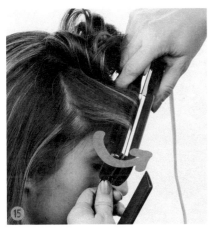 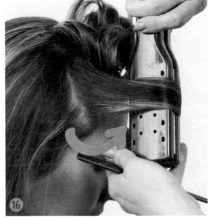 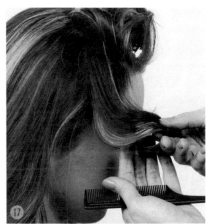

15 Move over to the right side above the ear. Curl a section with the flat iron curl, this time directing the curl forward toward the face.

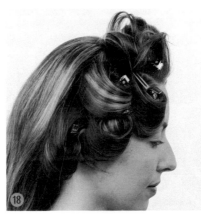 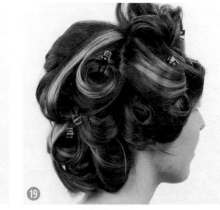

16 The iron is stationary while you run it along the hair shaft and rotate it.

17 Use your hands to form the piece into a stand-up pin curl while it is still warm and clip the hair to cool in this shape.

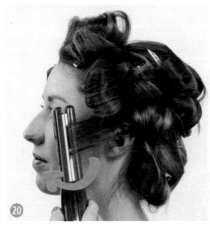 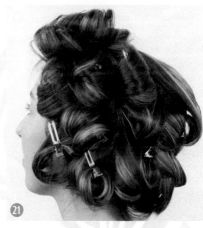

18 Curl the last of the hair the same on this side.

19 Use the same direction toward the face to curl the back of the head on the right side.

20 On the left side above the ear, repeat steps 15-17 with the curls directed around the left side of the face.

21 Finish the left half of the back of the head with the same curl directed around toward the left side of the face and clip the curls to cool.

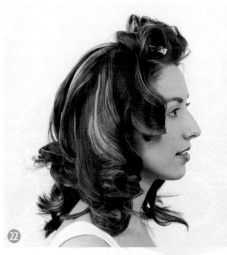

22 Remove the clips from the curls after they have cooled.

23 Brush the hair at the back of the hairstyle down and then forward toward the shoulder.

24 Comb the hair on the right side backward at the scalp.

25 When you have passed the ear, use your finger to press the hair against the scalp to hold it in position. Turn the direction of the comb around toward the chin.

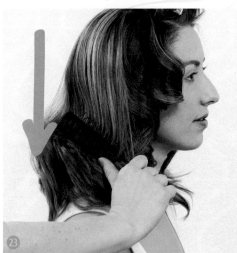

26 Finish combing this section around toward the chin to create a c-shape around the ear. Repeat these steps on the left side. Then, using your finger, press the side so the left hair above the ear lays tightly against the scalp and direct the hair back with pressure to accumulate behind the ear. Grip pin to secure.

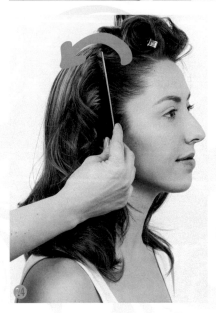 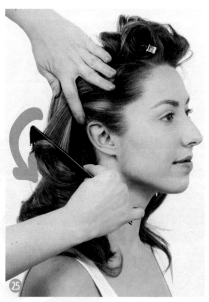 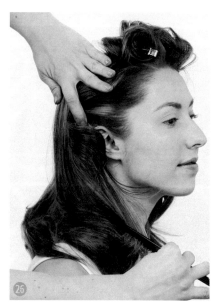

27 Comb out the hair above the forehead over to the right side. Once the comb has passed the right peak of the eyebrow, use your finger to press the hair and hold it in position.

28 Turn the direction of the comb down and forward toward the eye.

29 Arrange the hair around the face to roll into itself.

30 Use decorative grip pins to help hold the hair's position.

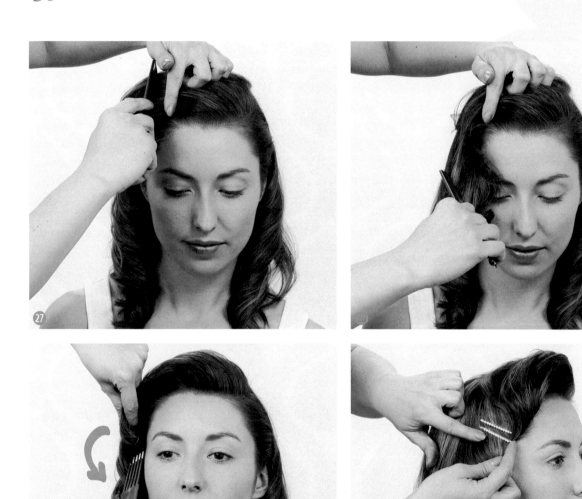

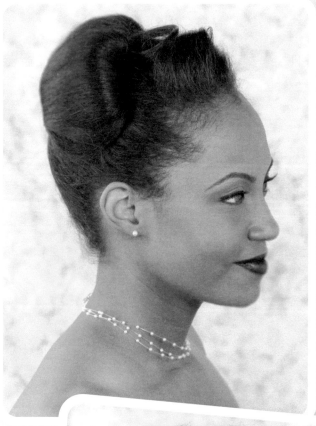

The inspiration for the **Lila** hairstyle comes from the elegant black-tie party scenes of movies from the 1940s. Perfect for an evening event, the Lila is both sophisticated and simple to create.

The silhouette gives the impression of a shape fanning out across the back of the crown. The design of the back can be paired with many different arrangements on the front.

The movement of the hair sweeping away from the cheeks accentuates the cheekbones and lifts the entire face.

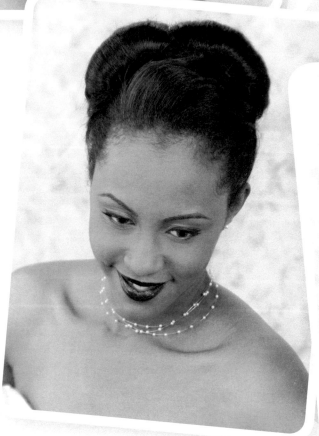

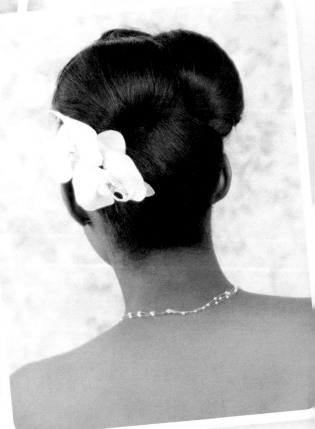

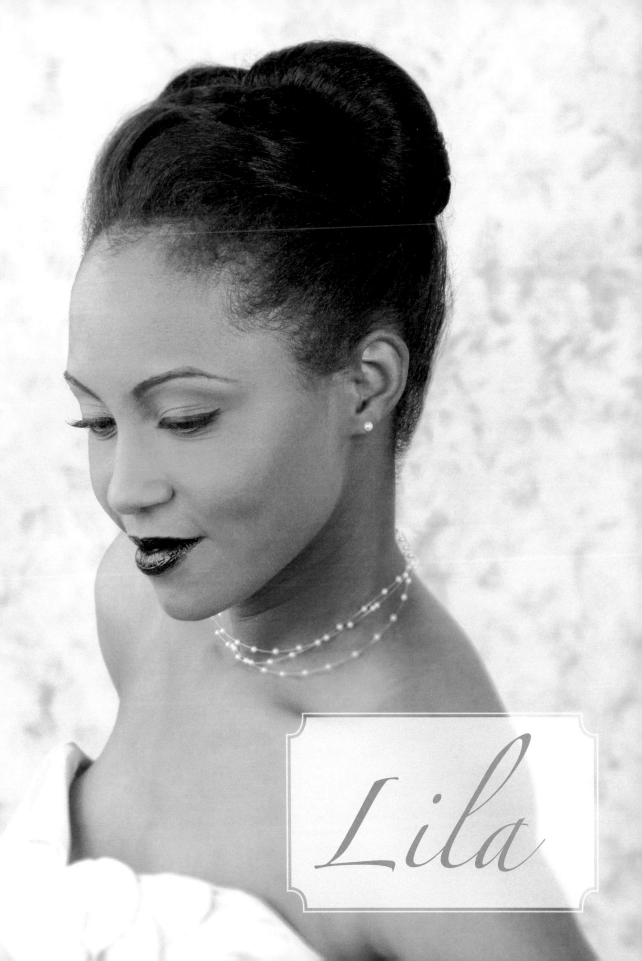

Lila

Supplies

thermal hair setting spray	carbon tail comb	ripple hair pins
hairspray	wide tooth comb	duckbill clips
pomade	loop and tail styling tool	small rubber bands
hot rollers	grip bob pins	hair filler

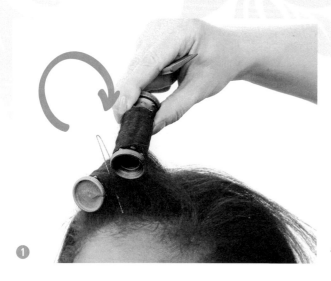

1 Prep using the steps described on page 22 for setting product into the hair. Use a volume blow-dry to eliminate any unruly growth patterns and add volume to the front hairline. Direction blow-dry as described on page 22 at the nape of the neck to avoid drooping at the hairline. Set a section of hair in small hot rollers directly above and perpendicular to the forehead.

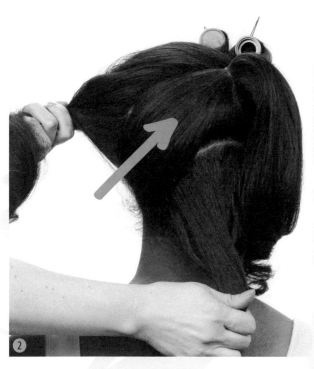

2 The Lila is created with 2 ponytails that are of equal height and sit at the back corners of the crown. To avoid visible parting lines, use the following technique to part the hair.

Imagine a diagonal section running around the center of the scalp beginning at the hairline in front of the right ear and going across to the left side of the nape of the neck. Part out a 4 inch wide section that follows this line and put it in a ponytail that sits toward the upper right side of the crown.

The hair for the second ponytail is made up of the hair below that includes everything running along the bottom hairline of the nape and the right of the nape. It also includes everything at the hairline in front of the left ear back to the top parting of the first ponytail.

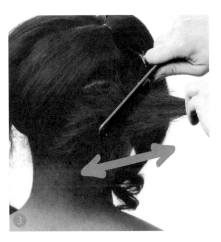 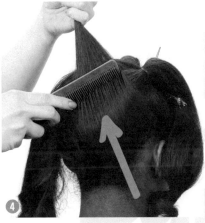 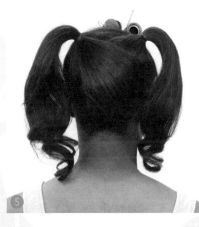

3 Back-comb the lower half of hair left to go in the second ponytail to lock the hairs together and add control.

4 Smooth the hairs and direct this section up to the left to be in line with the first ponytail. Bring all of the section together and secure with a small rubber band.

5 At this point all of the hair is either in the hot rollers set at the front in the first step or in one of the 2 ponytails. Notice the clean look with no visible parts.

6 Using the loop and tail tool, insert the tail back between the scalp and the rubber band of the right ponytail. Center the ponytail inside the loop.

7 Pull the tail all the way through along with the ponytail to create a topsytail twist.

8 Repeat steps 6 and 7 with the left ponytail.

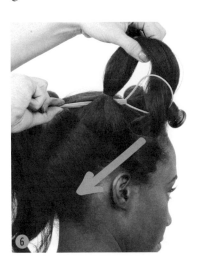 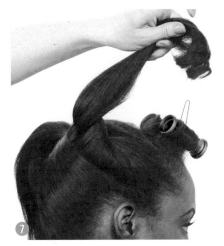 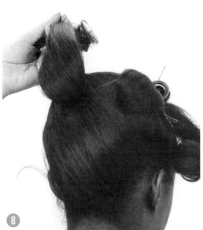

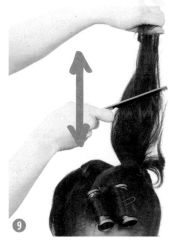

9 Hold the left ponytail straight up from the scalp and back-comb it to lock the hairs together. Smooth the other side with the comb.

10 For this hairstyle you will want 2 small, oblong hair fillers. See page 24 for a description of creating your own hair fillers.

11 Beginning with the ends of the ponytail, wrap the hair filler down toward the base in a semi-tight roll.

12 At the base, fan the edges of this new roll out to meet the scalp. Grip pin the roll and edges down to secure it.

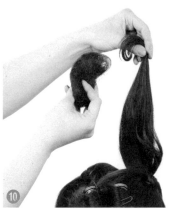

13 Repeat steps 9-12 on the ponytail on the right side. Back-comb the ponytail to lock the hair together and smooth the visible portion with the comb.

14 Roll a small, oblong hair filler down to the base.

15 At the base, fan the edges of this new roll out to meet the scalp. Grip pin the roll and edges down to secure it.

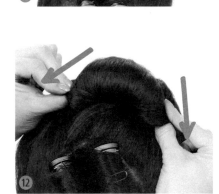

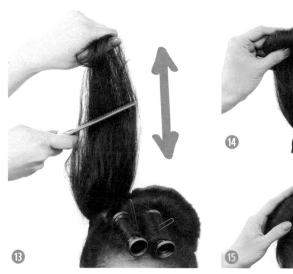

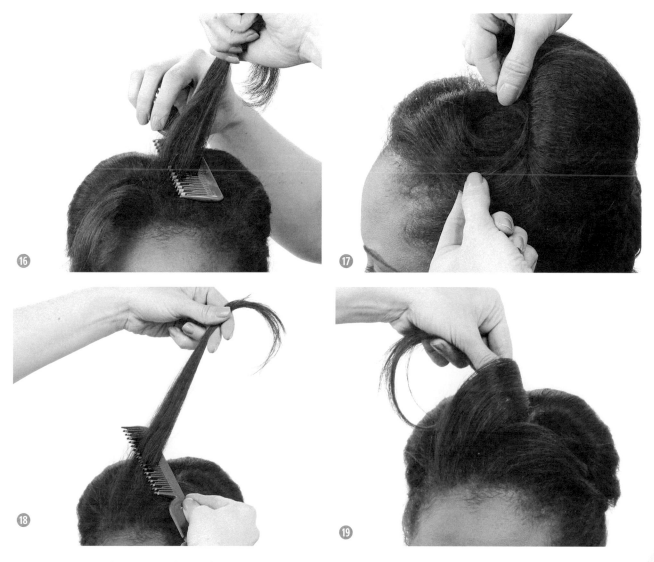

16 Remove the hot rollers from the front section. Working in small pieces, comb and back-comb the section to add volume and lock the hairs together.

17 Arrange the pieces in waves and pin curls.

18 Continue to comb and back-comb each piece until finished.

19 Arrange everything in overlapping sections.

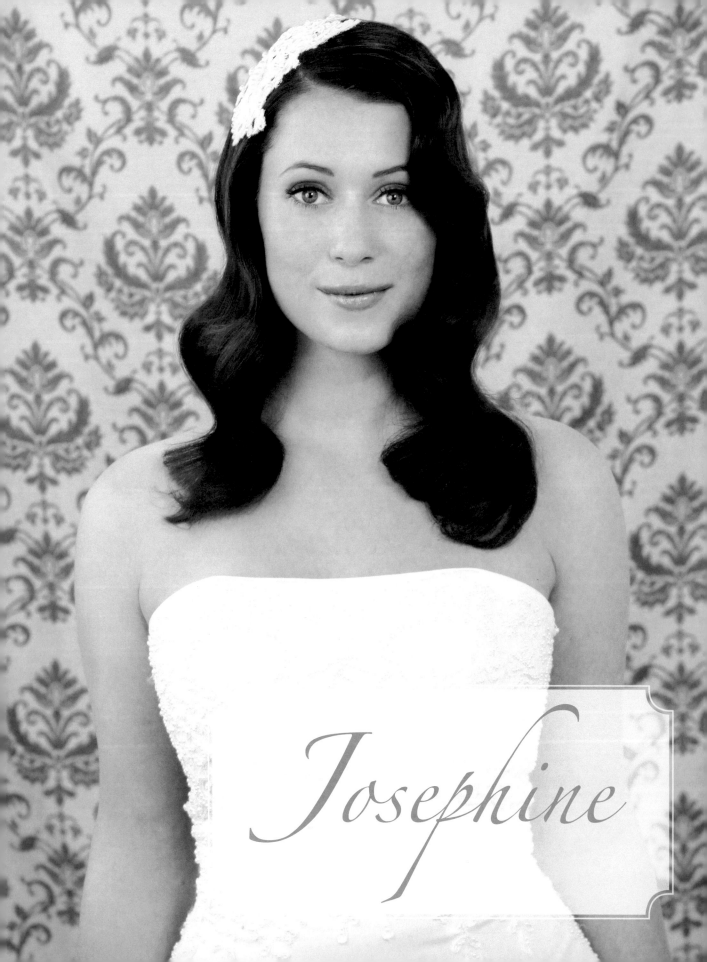

Josephine

The look of the **Josephine** is a highly requested vintage event hairstyle. The peek-a-boo bang reminiscent of 1940s actress Veronica Lake makes a woman feel flirty and sultry. This is a beautiful hairstyle that makes every woman look youthful.

Before committing to this hairstyle for an event, it is important to consider a couple important factors.

Hair that is all one length works best for this style. This hairstyle does not work great on hair that has layers. A key element to the hair laying in its waves is that they are equal to each other and actually confine each other to keep the wave pattern in place. Layers separate easily and mess up the uniformity.

The hair should hold curl well. The weight of the hair and the events of the day will slowly pull the curl looser. If hair doesn't hold a curl well, an option like the Ella hairstyle might be better suited. It uses a stronger curl and contains the hair a little better for longevity.

Last, consider that a photograph of a hairstyle and living in a hairstyle for a few hours can look like 2 different things. This hairstyle will move as you move and you may need to stay on top of it with a comb to keep the waves picture perfect.

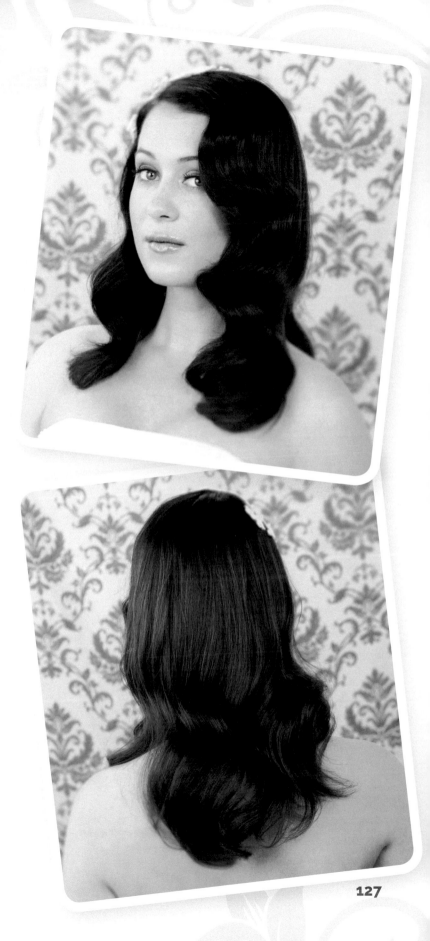

Supplies

thermal hair setting spray
hairspray
pomade
hair dryer

1¼ - ¾" tapered curling iron
1" curling iron
carbon tail comb
teaser brush

grip bob pins
duckbill clips
hair clips

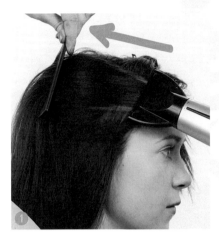 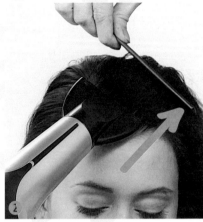 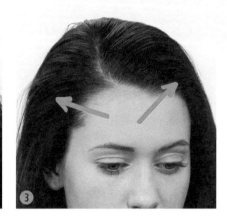

1 Prep using the steps described on page 22 for setting product into the hair. Part the hair above the outer corner of the right eyebrow. Using the steps described on page 23, base direction blow-dry the hair below the part back.

2 Base direction blow-dry the hair above the part diagonally back and to the left.

3 The hair should fan back and out from the part.

4 Separate a 1 inch thick piece from the left of the part and going back 4 inches from the front hairline and clip it off to the side for future styling. With the rest of the hair, working in 1x1 inch section, use the larger 1¼ - ¾" tapered curling iron to curl.

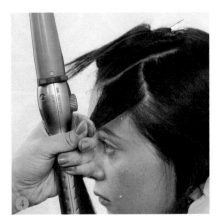 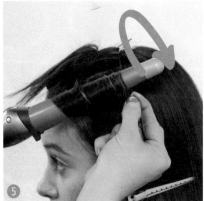 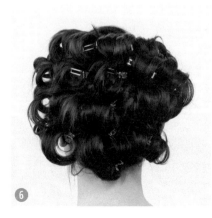

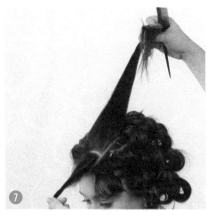

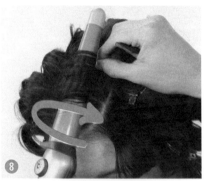

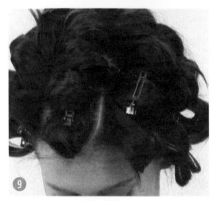

5 Curl using the right wrap pattern described on page 20. Keep the base sizes of each curl consistent in size and shape.

6 Curl in rows parallel to the floor all the way around to the other side of the head. Clip the curls to cool.

7 You should still have the small section clipped from step 4. Separate it into 1x1 inch pieces.

8 Curl using the right wrap pattern from page 20.

9 This section on the top will also be styled separate from the rest of the hairstyle.

10 Beginning at the bottom, remove the clips and brush the hair straight down toward the floor using a teaser brush. The teaser brush will help align the waves.

11 Continue brushing everything except the final row of curls from steps 7-8.

12 With all of the hair being curled uniformly, the wave around the head is also uniform.

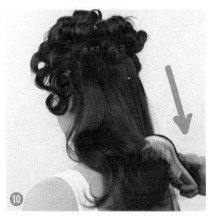

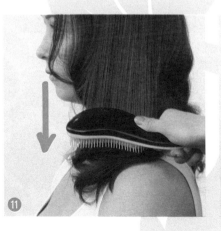

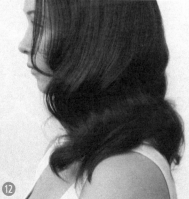

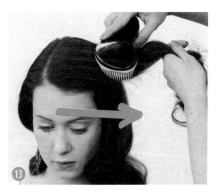
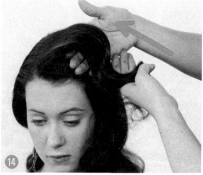
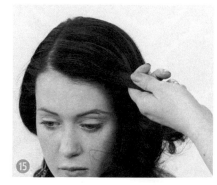

Creating a Marcel Wave

A true Marcel wave starts with a straight piece of hair. It can be hard to master and so I have developed a method that gives you a jump-start for faster results. Practice the motions with a cool iron to get the hang of it first. When you are ready, turn the curling iron to a medium setting. The iron should not be too hot.

13 Remove the clips from the final section of hair from steps 7-8. Brush it out in one piece using the teaser brush.

14 Release some tension in the hold allowing the wave to bounce back slightly and you will see the ridges and waves. You will use the curling iron to add some definition to these ridges.

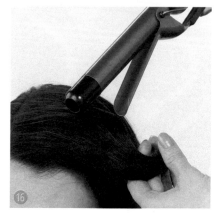

15 Section off a piece that is a little less than 2 inches wide and hold it in your left hand loose enough to make out the wave in the hair.

16 Hold a 1" curling iron in your right hand parallel to the floor with the shell facing down toward the shoulder. Open the shell.

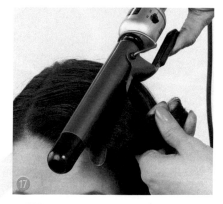

17 Slip the hair between the tongs, shell underneath and wand on top. The edge of the shell closest to you should align with the under side of the top ridge.

18 Close the iron. Roll the closed iron forward for a half turn, thereby rolling the hair up gently over the shell. Unroll the iron back to position 17 and remove the curling iron and you will see the ridge is more defined.

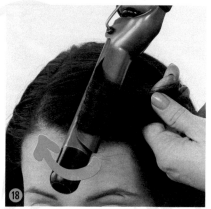

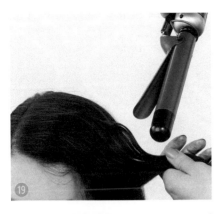
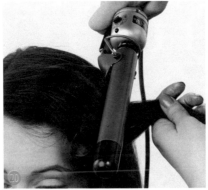
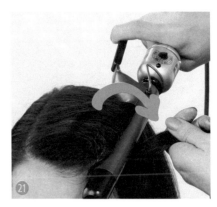

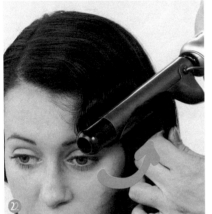

19 Turn the curling iron a quarter turn toward you.

20 Slip the hair between the tongs, shell underneath and wand on top. The edge of the shell at the top should align with the under side of the same ridge.

21 Close and roll the iron down for a quarter turn, thereby rolling the hair gently over the shell. Unroll the iron back to position 20 and remove the curling iron and you will see the ridge is more defined.

22 Move down to the ridge below and repeat steps 15-22 to define this next ridge.

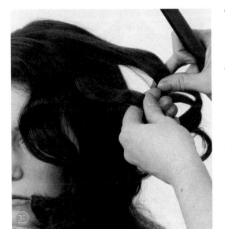

23 Take a 1 inch section at the back of this marceled piece and connect it with a 1 inch section of the top wave that has not yet been marceled.

24 Holding the hair gently, allow the waves to line up.

25 Repeat steps 13-22 until the top section of hair has a finished Marcel wave. If there is still some time before the event, use a hair net or snood to encase the curls and keep them off the neck until later.

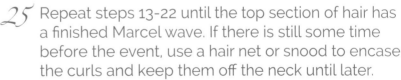

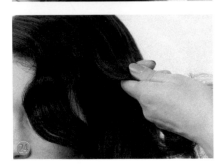
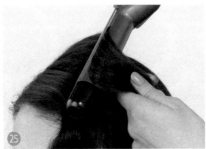
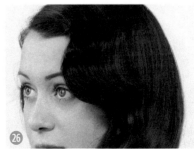

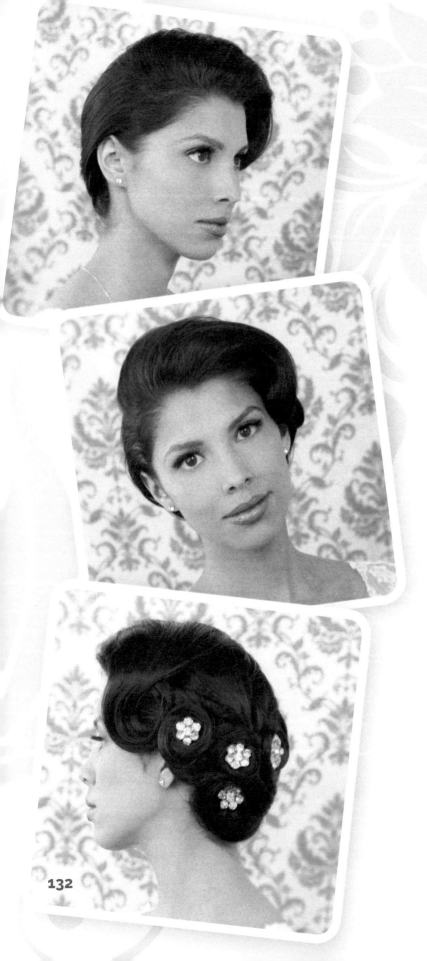

Dry pin curls can be used for many mid-20th century inspired hairstyles. Then they were the basic building block for creating curl. Now they are a common style technique for creating the texture of a vintage hairstyle.

In the 1950s, women often cropped their hair very short behind the neck. The dry pin curls of the **Cora** hairstyle keeps the hair close to the scalp to copy that silhouette. Volume over the forehead mimics the pompadour of the decade.

The volume over the forehead also serves another important purpose. In any bridal hairstyle, always consider the photographs of the day. For photographs that will be taken facing the camera, all the beautiful intricate detailing of the back will not show. The front of the hairstyle should capture the vintage feel as well for a cohesive look from every angle.

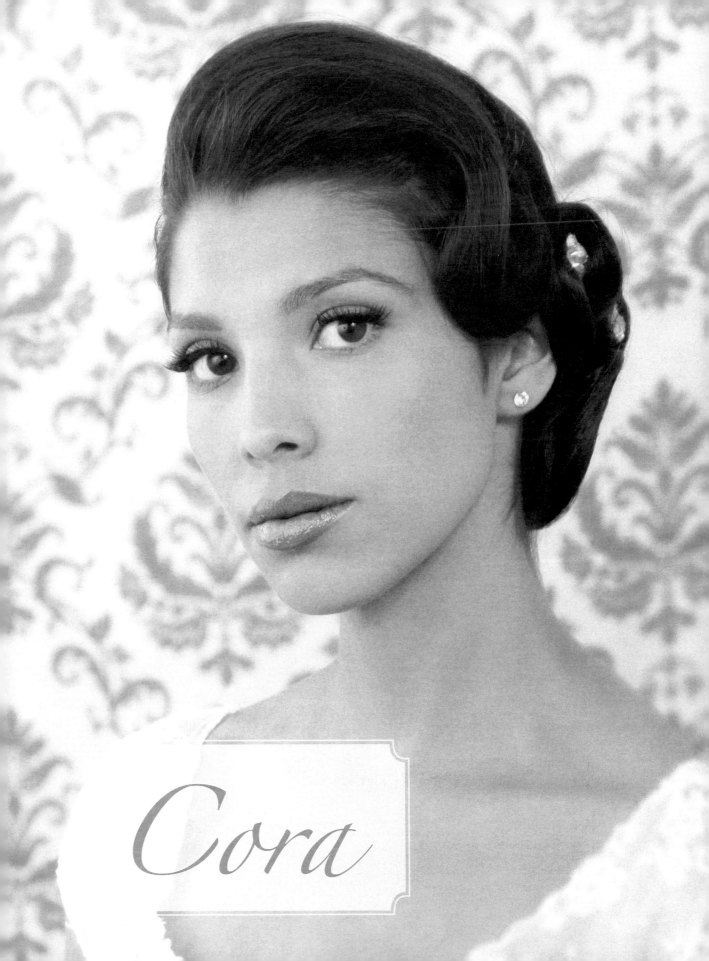

Cora

Supplies

volume spray
thermal hair setting spray
hairspray
pomade
hair dryer

1" curling iron
carbon tail comb
styling brush
grip bob pins
ripple hair pins

duckbill clips
hair clips
2 ¾" plastic craft needle
lightweight monofilament

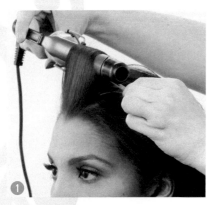

1 Prep using the steps described on page 22 for setting product into the hair. Use a volume blow-dry to eliminate any unruly growth patterns and add volume to the front hairline. Curl all of the hair with the 1" curling iron.

2 Curl everything in a brick-lay pattern on-base for volume. Clip the hair to cool. Remove the clips after cooled and part above the right eyebrow.

3 The Cora is built from the bottom up in several small sections. First part out the lower area below the occipital bone.

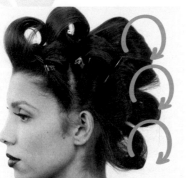

4 On the left side, take a 2 inch wide section and comb it straight up and flat against the scalp.

5 Pin with a large grip pin to hold it flat for the time being.

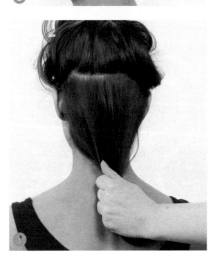

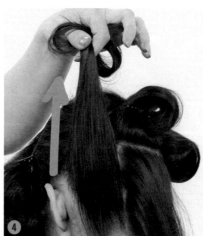

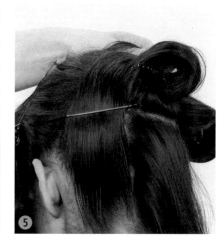

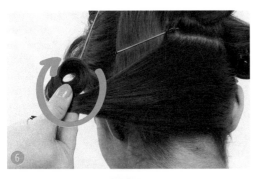

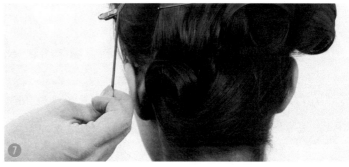

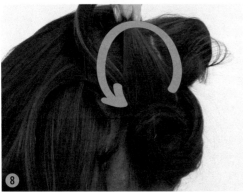

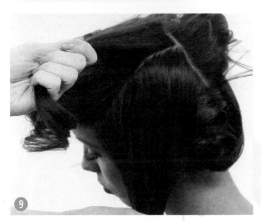

6 Using the second piece of this lower section on the right. Comb it over to the left so that the base lays flat against the scalp. Sculpt the ends into a dry pin curl and place the pin curl so that it sits on top of the base of the section to its left. Use a little pomade on your fingers for control and to add shine while you work.

7 To avoid visible grip pins, use the plastic craft needle and monofilament thread to secure the pin curls in this hairstyle. See page 26 for a description of steps in hair sewing.

8 Remove the large grip pin holding the section from step 4. Form the ends of this section into a dry pin curl and arrange and secure it just above the pin curl from step 6 using hair sewing.

9 The next section is created parting a line from behind the left ear up 2 inches and then forward to the front hairline. Comb the base of this section down and slightly forward toward the chin. Part a second piece that is 2x2 inches directly above it and toward the back of the crown.

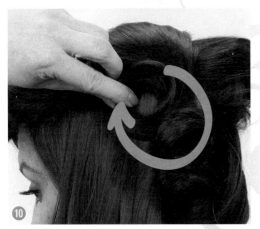

10 Form this second section into a dry pin curl and arrange it over the base of the first section below it. Secure it with grips pins or sew it to secure it.

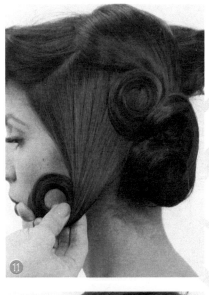

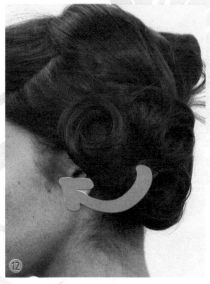

11 Form the ends of the lower section into a dry pin curl.

12 Secure it over its base with grip pins or hair sewing. All of the hair on the left side of the head should now be up and secure in the hairstyle. That leaves a section above the forehead and a small section on the right and back of the head.

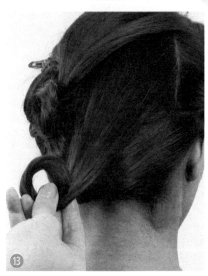

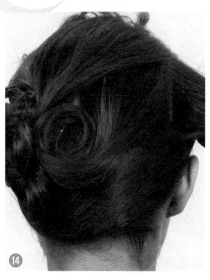

13 Work your way back over to the back of the head. With the small section that sits on the occipital bone, form a dry pin curl.

14 Secure the pin curl with hair sewing or grip pins.

15 Move to the right side of the head. At the top of the right side section, create a diagonal parting that graduates slightly up. The final hairstyle should not have visible parts and this will help later to hide it.

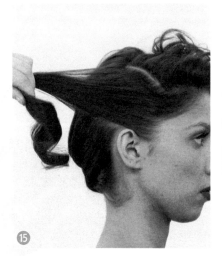

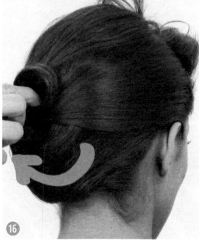

16 Comb the ends of this right section around the back and form into a dry pin curl. Secure with hair sewing or grip pins.

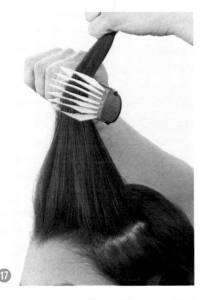

17 With the final section above the forehead brush the hair out.

18 Back-comb the base to add volume. Continue to back-comb up the hair shaft to lock the hairs together.

19 Bring the hair over to the left side of the head. Smooth the top and use the comb to fan the hair over the top of the crown.

20 Comb and shape the ends of the piece to the left of the temple.

21 Arrange the ends to create a peek-a-boo shaped pin curl that sits loosely on the left. Grip pin or sew the piece to secure.

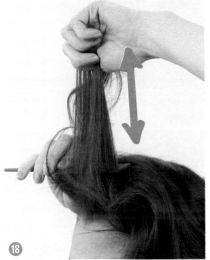

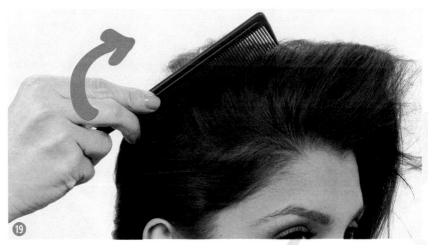

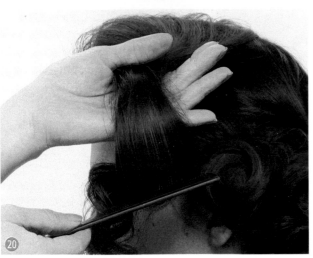

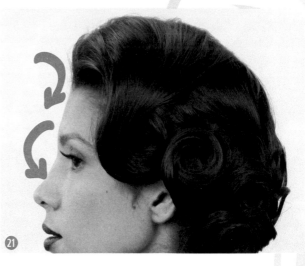

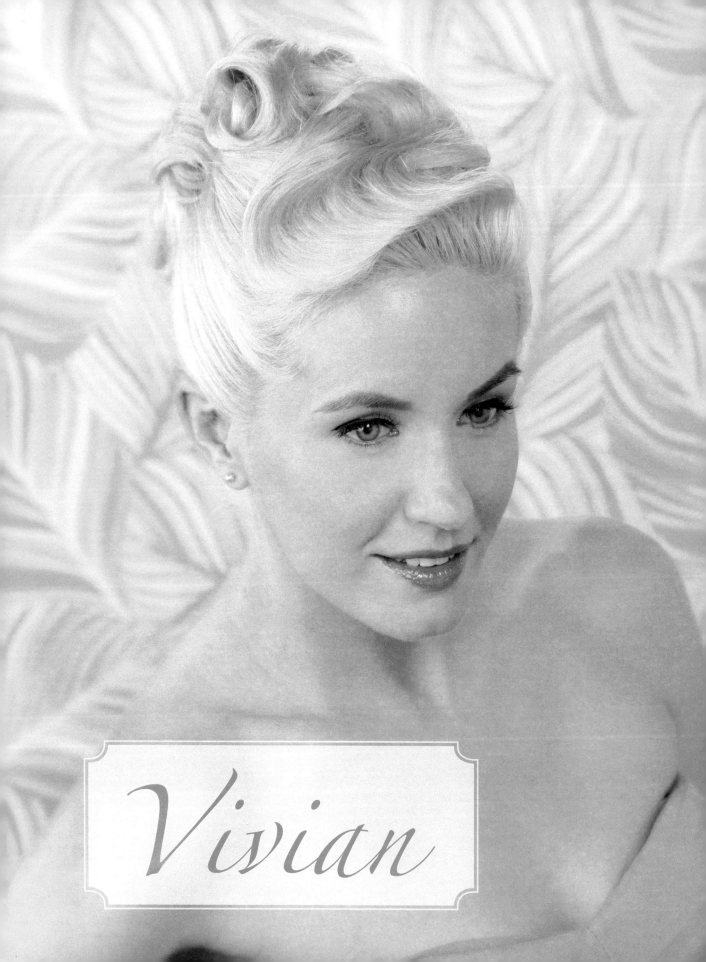

Vivian

The deep wave at the hairline in the **Vivian** hairstyle was a detail used for many years. Although this hair style is amongst the 1950s inspired looks, the treatment at the front would easily go along with a 1930s or 1940s inspired hairstyle.

It is created with a water-wave, but instead of using your fingers to form the wave and setting under a hooded hair dryer for 40 minutes, a comb and hand held hair dryer are all you need.

Practice this technique a few times and always remember, with wet hair, it will dry in whatever shape you dry it in. Once it is set, there is no changing it.

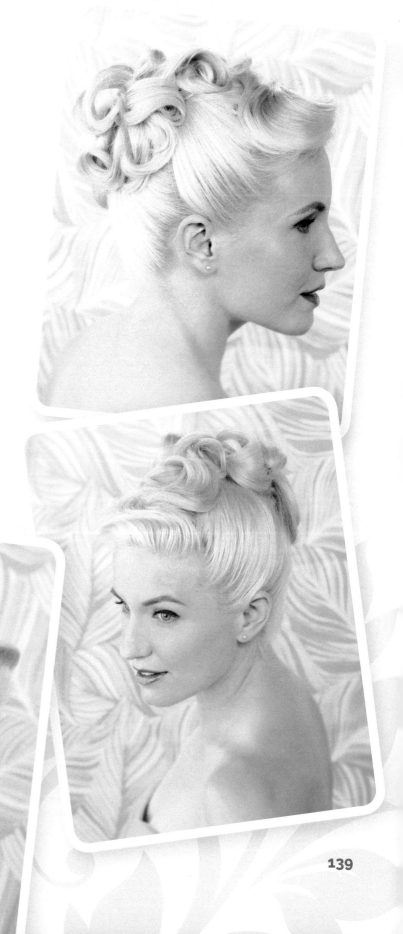

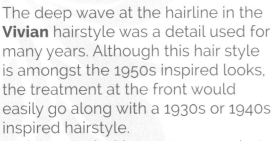

Supplies

spray bottle with water
thermal hair setting spray
hairspray
pomade
hair dryer

hair dryer diffuser
  attachment
hot rollers
carbon tail comb
carbon cutting comb

grip bob pins
ripple hair pins
duckbill clips
hair clips
small rubber bands

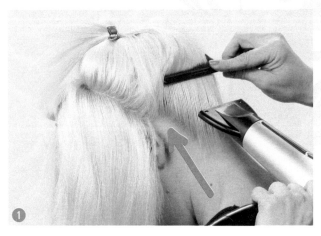

1 Prep using the steps described on page 22 for setting product into the hair. Base direction blow-dry at the nape of the neck and around the hairline by the ears to avoid droops at the hairline. See page 23 for more on base direction.

2 Create a high sitting ponytail that is slightly to the left using all of the hair on the back of the head from the crown down to the nape of the neck. Secure it with a rubber band using the steps on page 27.

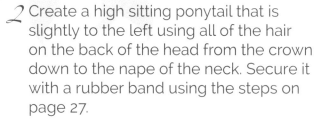

3 Create a second ponytail that is slightly off center to the right.

4 The hair for this ponytail comes from the sides of the head and the apex of the crown.

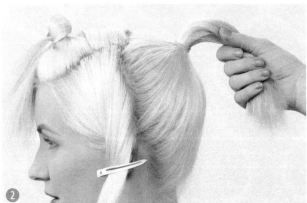

5 The final section is above the forehead and is 2 inches deep.

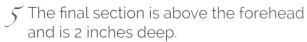

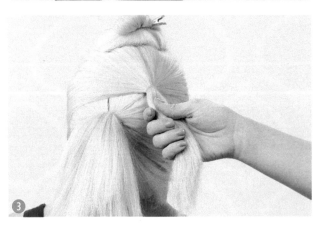

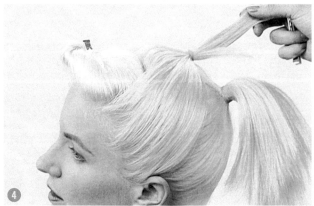

6 Wet down the base, but not the ends of the hair.

7 Comb it back with a carbon cutting comb to smooth all of the hair.

8 Hold the comb in your left hand and the hair dryer with nozzle in your right hand. Insert the wide tooth side of the comb at the hairline and comb back in an arch to the left an inch or so.

9 Without moving the position of your hand, gently dig the teeth of the comb down into the scalp hair pressing the teeth forward and thereby pressing volume into the front of the hairline.

10 Dry while pressing a wave and ridge into the hairline by pressing the hair dryer nozzle and comb together. Also use the air speed of the hair dryer at an angle to force an arch into the hair.

11 Work across the hairline in strokes going left and right.

12 Duckbill clip to hold.

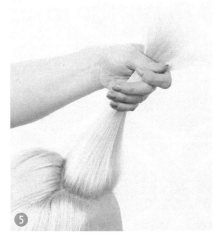

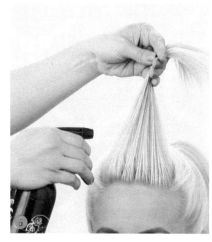

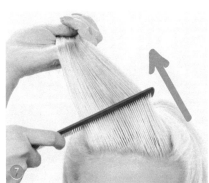

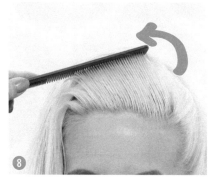

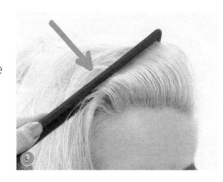

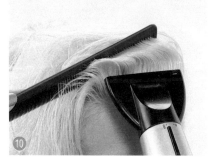

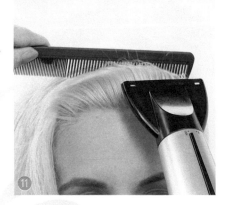

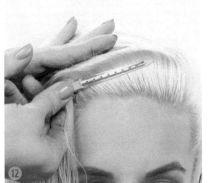

13 Insert the wide tooth side of the comb behind the ridge you have just created. With gentle pressure comb back in a wave pattern, first to toward the right ear.

14 Arch the comb's pattern then to the left to form an arched dip in the surface of the hair.

15 Use the teeth of the comb to hold the hair stationary. With the nozzle of the hairdryer pointing into the arch at an angle, dry the hair in the center of the arch.

16 Without removing the teeth of the comb from the hair, use your finger to press the arch against the scalp. Leaving your hand with the comb in its position, rotate the comb teeth back away from the front hairline.

17 Gently press the comb teeth down for pressure into the base and rotate the teeth back toward the front hairline grabbing the hair.

18 Shift the comb forward defining the arch more and enhancing a second ridge behind it.

19 Dry the ridge pressing the comb and dryer nozzle together to define it.

20 Duckbill clip the waves and ridges to hold.

21 Use the diffuser attachment on the hair dryer and finish drying any spots that may still be damp.

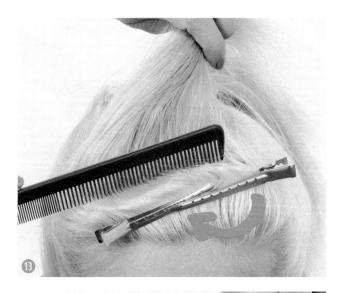

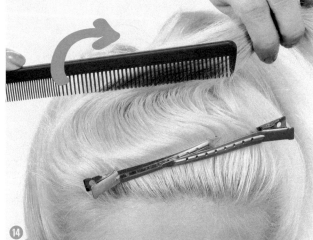

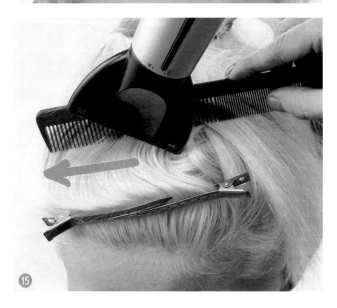

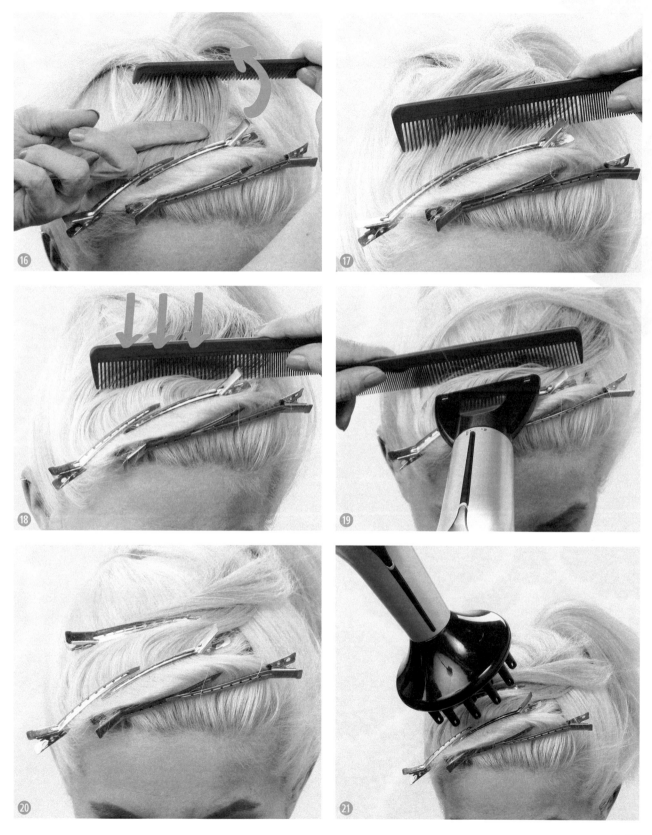

143

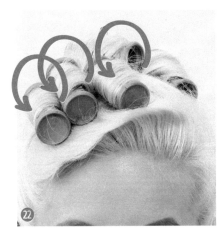

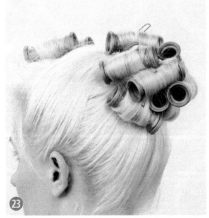

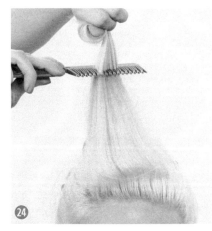

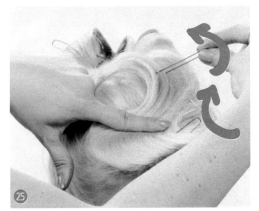

22 Set the ends of this top section in small hot rollers rolled toward the right ear.

23 Roll all the ends of the 2 ponytails in small hot rollers.

24 After the rollers have cooled, remove them and comb out the top section.

25 Arrange the wave and position it with ripple pins.

26 Insert small grip pins to secure the wave. Remove the ripple pins.

27 Finish arranging the top section of hair and grip pin to secure.

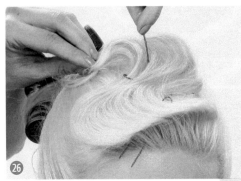

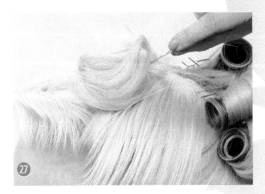

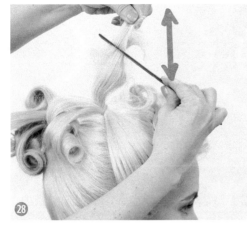

28 Remove the rest of the hot rollers. Back-comb one curl from the forward most ponytail to lock the hairs together.

29 Smooth the hairs with a comb and arrange the curl to cover the rubber band around the ponytail. Use ripple pins to hold the curl in place temporarily. This will make it easier to change your arrangement if needed before the hairstyle is permanently secured in place.

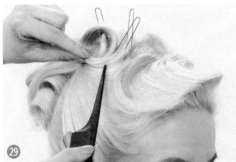

30 Back-comb a second curl to lock the hairs together and smooth the hairs with a comb.

31 Arrange the curl around the ponytail base.

32 Continue this with each piece until the curls are all arranged in the desired formation.

33 Add grip pins wherever ripple pins are holding to secure everything. Remove all the ripple pins.

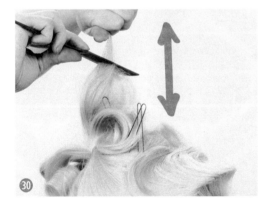

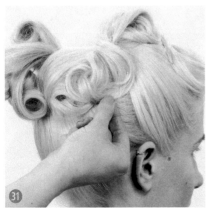

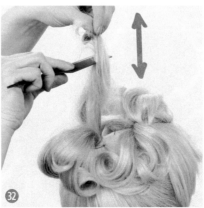

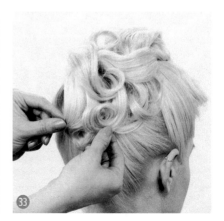

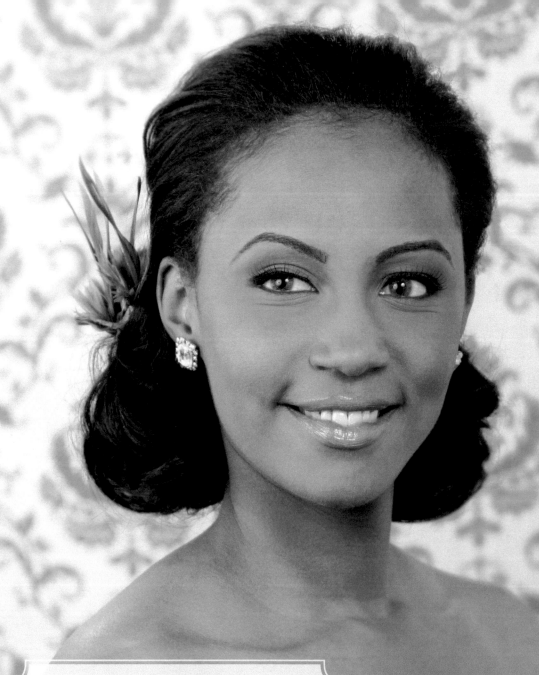

Grace

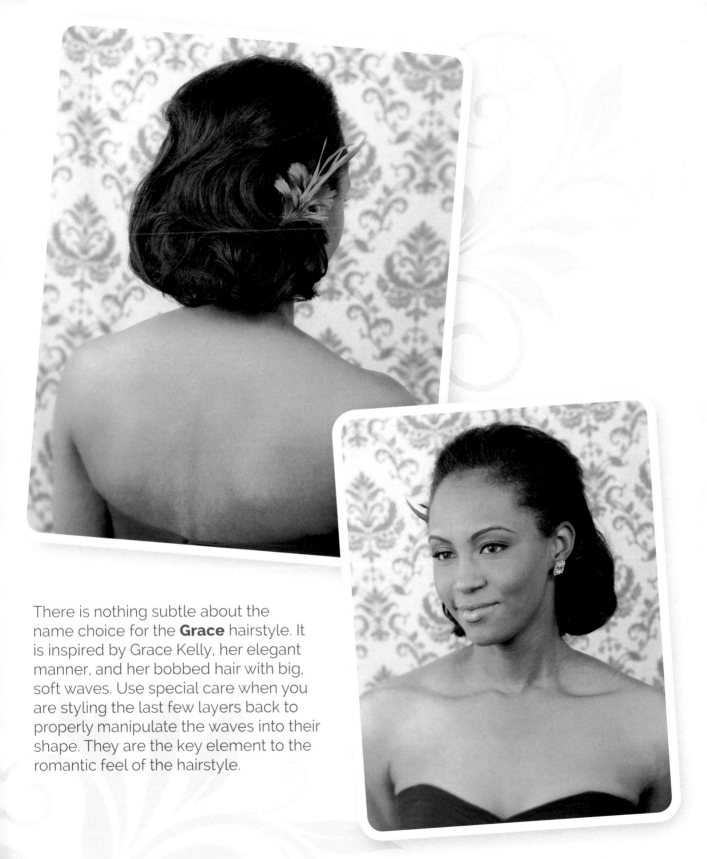

There is nothing subtle about the name choice for the **Grace** hairstyle. It is inspired by Grace Kelly, her elegant manner, and her bobbed hair with big, soft waves. Use special care when you are styling the last few layers back to properly manipulate the waves into their shape. They are the key element to the romantic feel of the hairstyle.

Supplies

volume spray
thermal hair setting spray
hairspray
pomade
hair dryer

¾" curling iron
carbon tail comb
wide tooth comb
round vent brush
grip bob pins

ripple hair pins
duckbill clips
hair clips
small rubber band

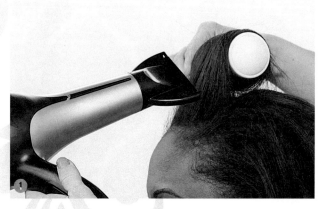

1 Prep using the steps described on page 22 for setting product into the hair. Use a volume blow-dry to eliminate any unruly growth patterns and add volume to the front hairline.

2 Set 4 or 5 on base small hot roller curls toward the top of the front hairline.

Using a ¾" curling iron, curl all the hair on the back of the head, but focus the curls toward the ends of the hair that fall below the nape of the neck. Clip the curls to cool.

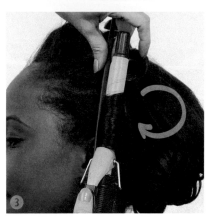

3 Hold the curling iron perpendicular to the floor and with the 2x2 inch section of hair above the ears. Curl the entire piece of hair toward the face. Keep a comb between the client's scalp and the curling iron for safety.

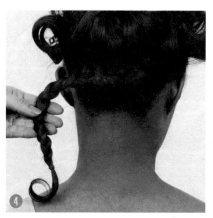

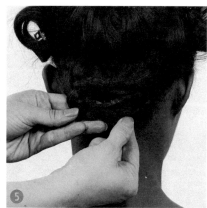

4 Part out a 2 inch deep section at the base of the neck. Braid the lower section across into a horizontal French braid and secure the end with a small rubber band.

5 Twist the end of the braid to overlap the scalp and use grip bob pins to secure it in a tight mass.

6 Row by row, start to take out the clips holding the curls.

7 With the first row, back-comb to lock the hairs together.

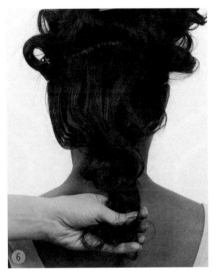
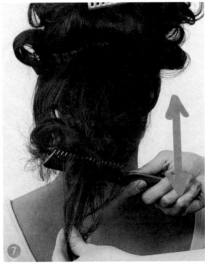
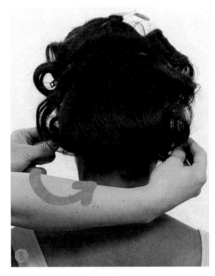

8 Rotate the ends under and grip pin them to the braid underneath to start the faux bob. Fan the edges out wider than the earlobes.

9 Let down another row of curls and finger through them to spread them around the back of the head.

10 Using ripple pins, gently secure the new layer to the layer beneath it toward the lower half at its bulkiest point.

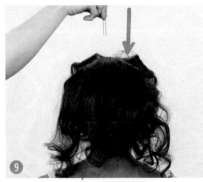
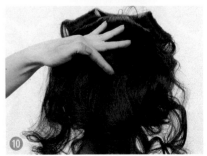

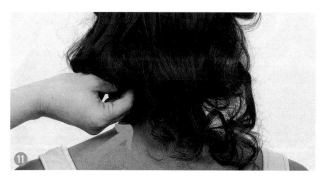
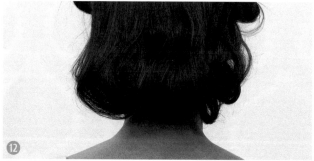

11 Back-comb the ends of the upper layer to lock the hairs together and turn the ends under.

12 Use grip bob pins to secure the ends to the braid underneath. Continue with the rest of the hair on the back of the head. Leave the side curls and the hot roller curls for the next steps.

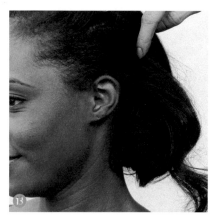
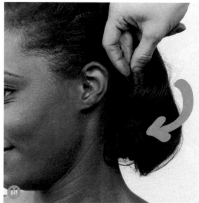
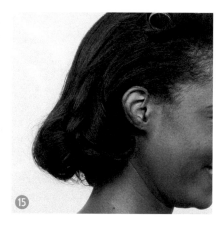

13 Use your finger to direct the base of the curl on the left side back into the mass of hair that has been accumulating behind the earlobe. Grip pin it to secure it back.

14 Arrange the ends of the curl to rotate together toward the ear. Grip pin it in place.

15 Repeat the same steps on the right side.

16 Remove the rear most hot rollers. Back-comb the section at the base to add volume.

17 Bring the piece back down over the back of the style and smooth the stray hairs on top. Arrange the wave of the hair with a wide tooth comb and ripple pins. Press the base of the section forward with the comb to maintain the volume,

18 Smooth the wave down the back of the hairstyle moving the comb left and right in a wave pattern.

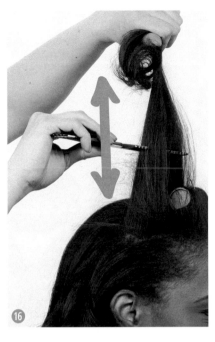

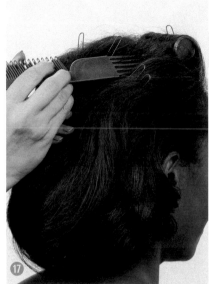

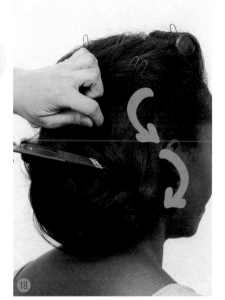

19. Pin with small grip pins to secure.

20. Remove the last of the hot rollers and back-comb the base for volume. Continue to back-comb up the hair shaft to lock the hairs together and spread the wave.

21. Bring the hair back over the hairstyle.

22. Smooth the stray hairs on top. Arrange the wave of the hair with a wide tooth comb. Smooth the wave down the back of the hairstyle moving the comb left and right in a wave pattern.

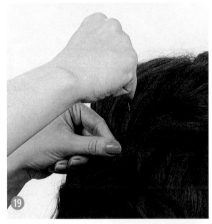

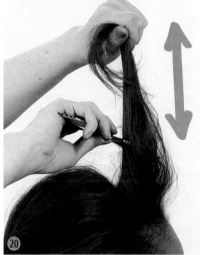

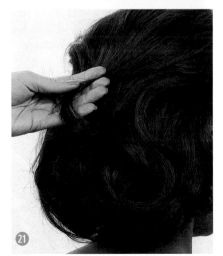

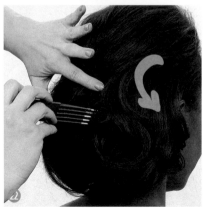

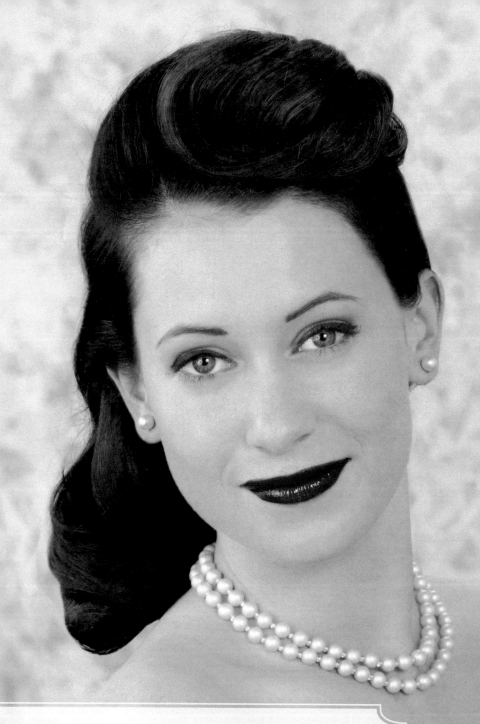

Constance

The **Constance** hairstyle is designed to add a little fun and whimsy to the party. The silhouette is a modern take on the form of the 1950s. While the back sweeps around the right of the face, the front of the hairstyle juts up and to the left in a swirling pompadour shape.

The design of the back is a very good option for someone who still wants to feel like their hair is down, but needs to keep it contained because it will lose its curl too quickly. The technique can be paired with other front design as well like the Ruby or Cora hairstyles.

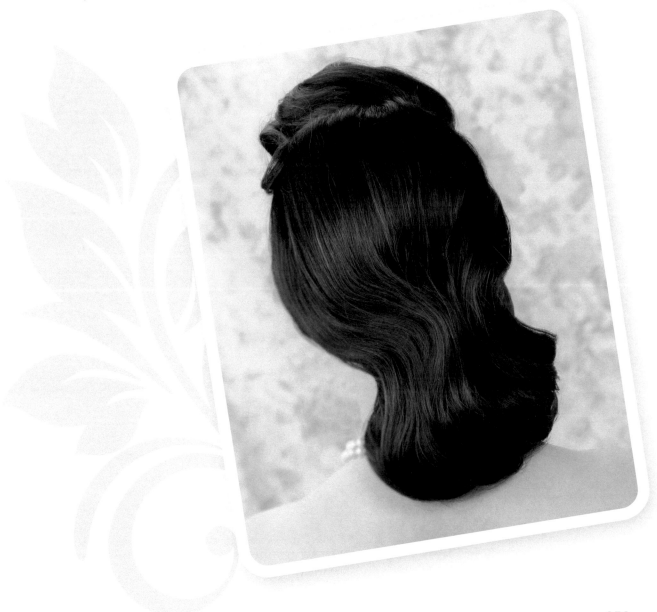

Supplies

thermal hair setting spray	carbon tail comb	ripple hair pins
hairspray	wide tooth comb	duckbill clips
pomade	styling brush	hair clips
1" curling iron	grip bob pins	hair net with elastic

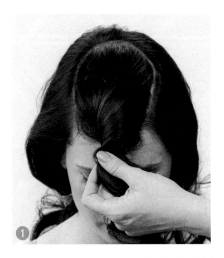

1 Prep using the steps described on page 22 for setting product into the hair. Use a volume blow-dry to eliminate any unruly growth patterns and add volume to the front hairline. Section out a horseshoe shaped area on top of the head.

2 Separate this into wide, slightly diagonal slices for curling. Use a 1" curling iron for on base curls.

3 Curl the top in consecutive curls that roll back.

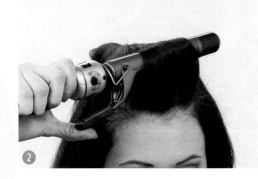

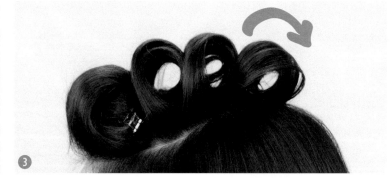

4 Turn the curling iron perpendicular with the floor.

5 Set the rest of the hair in barrel curls rotating to the right around the horseshoe section on top. Curl a second row below at the nape of the neck also rotating right.

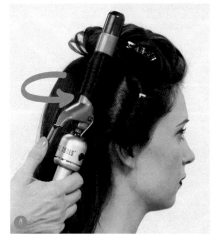

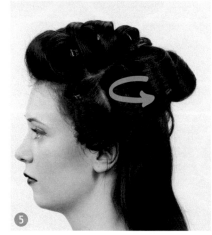

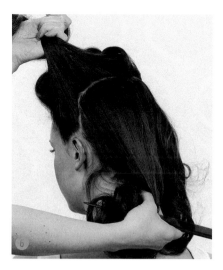
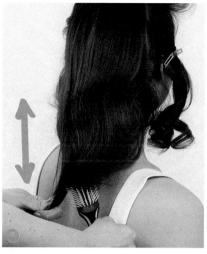
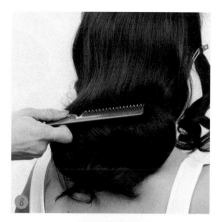

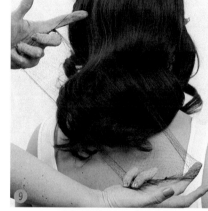

6 Leave the top section clipped in its curls. Draw a part that runs from behind the left ear, up above the occipital bone and over in an upside down horseshoe shape ending behind the right ear.

7 Back-brush this entire portion to lock the hairs together and spread the shape.

8 Smooth the hairs over the top with a comb.

9 Use a bouffant sized hairnet with elastic in a color that matches the hair.

10 Wrap the hairnet around the bottom of the hair mass to encase it. Pull the right edge of the hair net up and to the right. This will direct the entire hair mass over to the right.

11 Use grip pins to secure it.

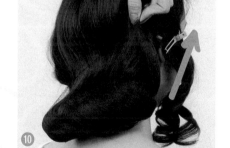

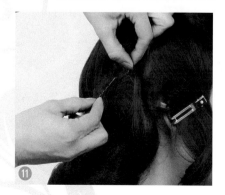

155

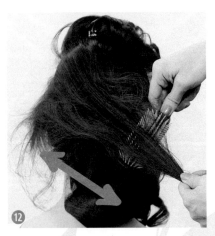 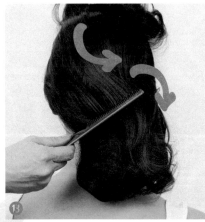 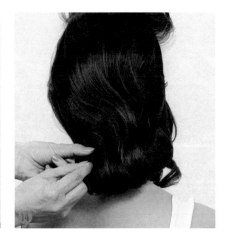

12 Bring down the rest of the hair that does not include the top section that is still clipped in its curls. Back-brush the hair directing it to the right as you do. This will lock the hairs together in a diagonal direction across the rear mass of hair in the hairnet.

13 Smooth over the top with a comb.

14 Press grip pins through the new layer down into the hair in the hairnet underneath to secure the layer. Wrap the ends under the hair mass underneath and secure them with grip pins. This would also be a good spot to sew the ends under to ensure they are secure for a long time. See page 26 for more information about hair sewing.

15 With the section of hair above the right ear, back-brush directing it back.

16 Comb and arrange the hair to wrap back forward over the front of the hair in the hairnet.

17 Use grip pins or hair sewing to secure it along behind the ear and forward over the hairnet.

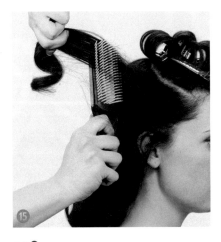 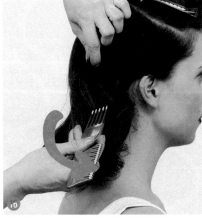 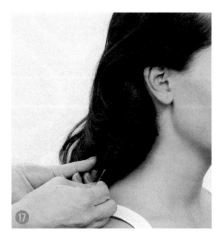

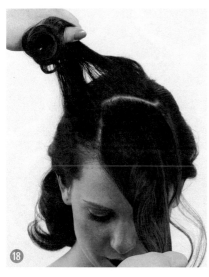

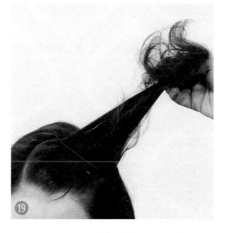

18 Remove the clips from the top curled section and separate as illustrated in image 18.

19 Brush the larger, square section back and to the left. Back-brush to lock the hairs together. Insert a large grip pin at the base to hold the base placement.

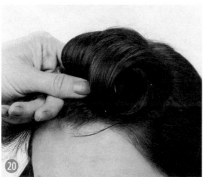

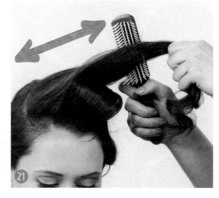

20 Roll the section beginning with the ends into a large, barrel roll on a slight diagonal to the right.

21 Using the rest of the hair, back-brush it while directing it around behind the barrel roll.

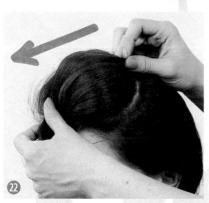

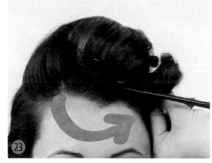

22 Lay it over the barrel to cover it.

23 Direct the rest of the piece under and to the left into a swoop.

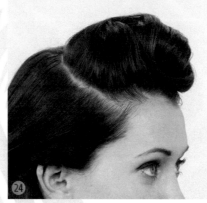

24 Arrange the hair for balance and design and grip pin everything in place to secure it. Use ripple pins as on page 28 to aid with style and hiding grip pins.

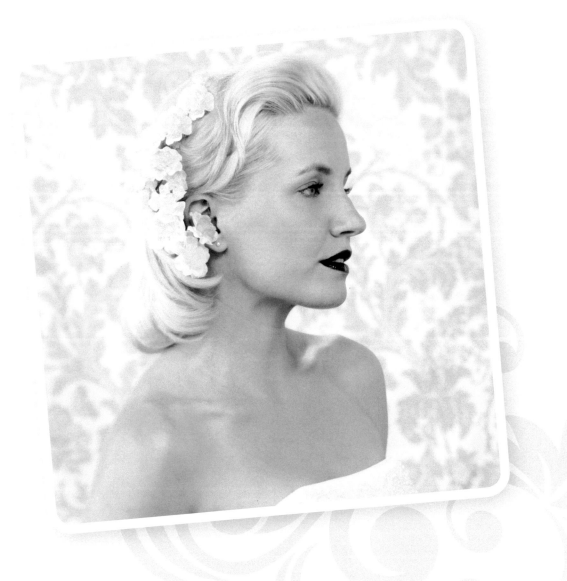

The **Kathryn** hairstyle is an interpretation of the pageboy hairstyle which has come in and out of fashion for many years. It was a popular style in the 1940s and into the 1950s.

Here it is designed to be well contained and above the shoulders so that it holds its shape for many hours. The texture of the style is smooth and simple, but the sophistication is very impactful.

In the 1940s, brides often decorated their hair along the sides and behind the ears with many little wax or fabric orange blossoms. The simplicity of the Kathryn hairstyle looks wonderful with lots of added texture from fabric flowers.

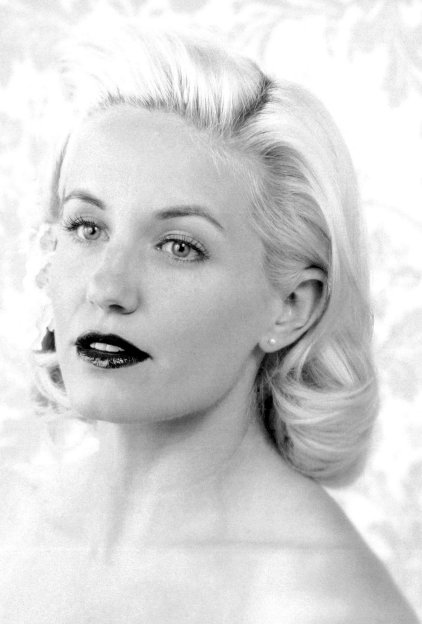

Kathryn

Supplies

thermal hair setting spray	hair dryer diffuser	ripple hair pins
hairspray	attachment	duckbill clips
pomade	carbon tail comb	hair clips
hot rollers	round vent brush	hair filler
hair dryer	grip bob pins	ribbon

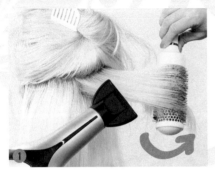

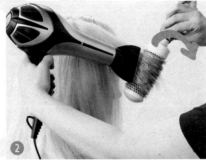

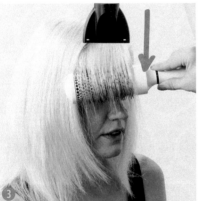

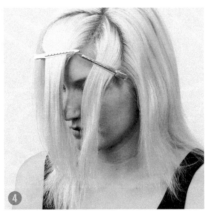

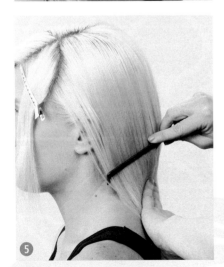

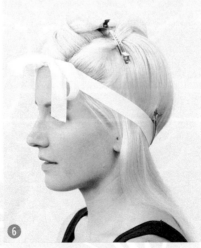

1. Prep steps for the Kathryn are similar to the steps for the Betty hairstyle. Prep using the steps described on page 22 for setting product, but use a round brush blow-dry directing the hair forward around the face.

2. Start at the lowest section working your way up always directing the hair around toward the face.

3. At the hairline, direct the hair over the forehead.

4. Part the hair above the left eyebrow. Separate 2 triangular sections on either side of the part.

5. Comb all of the rest of the hair tightly against the back of the head and down the nape of the neck.

6 The next step requires a wide ribbon or rolled up scarf. Either will be fine. Center it at the center of the nape of the neck over the hair. Tie it around the forehead snuggly. Use duckbill clips to keep it from slipping. The 2 triangular sections on top should be left out for the next step.

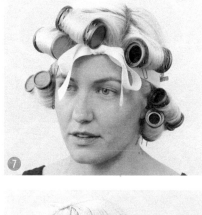

7 Roll these 2 triangular sections in large hot rollers set forward over the ribbon/scarf.

8 Set the ends of the hair hanging below the ribbon/scarf in the back in small hot rollers. Heat the back up with the hair dryer diffuser attachment and then allow it to cool to help set the indentation and curls.

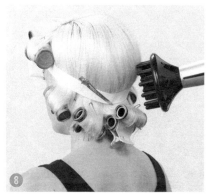

9 Let everything cool and remove the ribbon/scarf and hot rollers. In sections beginning at the bottom and working your way up, back-comb the ends of the hair.

10 Work around the lower level back-combing the ends, locking them together and creating a fan effect that travels from shoulder to shoulder around the back.

11 Smooth over the top lightly with a comb to line the hairs up and improve the appearance, Lightly spray with hairspray.

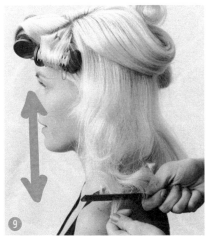
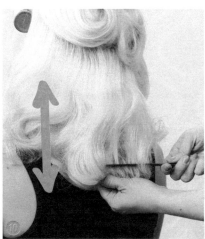
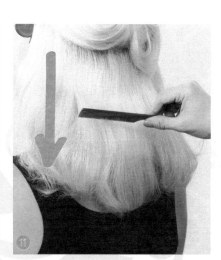

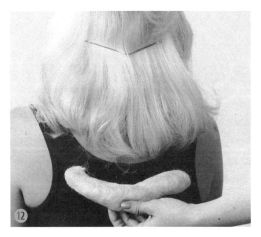

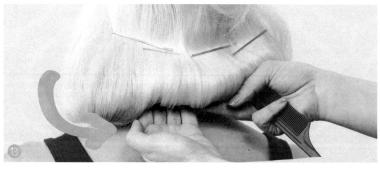

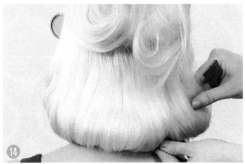

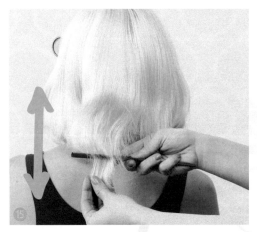

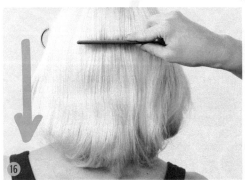

12 Insert large grip pins across the middle to help hold the fanning form. This step requires a hair filler in a cylindrical shape that is just long enough to stretch from behind the ear of one side and over to behind the other ear.

13 Roll the ends and the hair filler up underneath the back until the form is level with the bottom of the neck.

14 Arrange the hair snuggly around the filler and use grip pins to secure everything. This would also be a good spot to sew the ends under to ensure they are secure for a long time. See page 26 for more information about hair sewing.

15 Lower down the upper section of hair over the back. Work around the lower level back-combing the ends, locking them together and creating a fan effect that travels from shoulder to shoulder around the back.

16 Smooth over the top lightly with a comb to line the hairs up and improve the appearance, Lightly spray with hairspray. Smooth the hair around and under the filler at the bottom and grip pin under if the hair is too long.

17 Comb the side to roll over the ear in a tapered bob. Grip pin any ends if the hair is too long.

18 Insert the teeth of the comb above the ear and gently comb back until you reach directly above the ear. This action brings the tapered bob roll up and perpendicular to the floor creating the page boy effect. Leave the comb at this point to hold the shape.

19 Use a decorative clip to secure the hair. Remove the comb. Repeat these steps on the opposite side.

20 Remove the hot rollers from the front hairline. Back-comb at the base to add volume. Bring the hair over to the side.

21 Massage the hair and run your fingers through at the hairline a little to add texture and lift to the front. Arrange the hair for balance and design. Use ripple pins as on page 28 to aid with style and hiding grip pins.

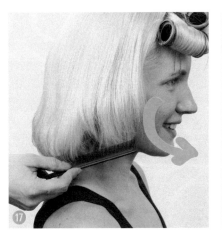
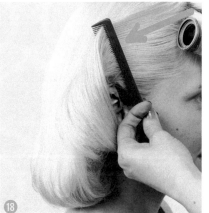
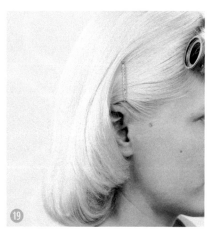

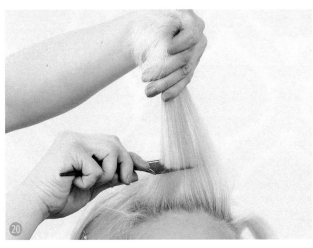
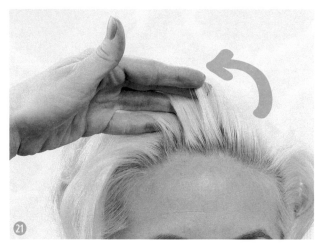

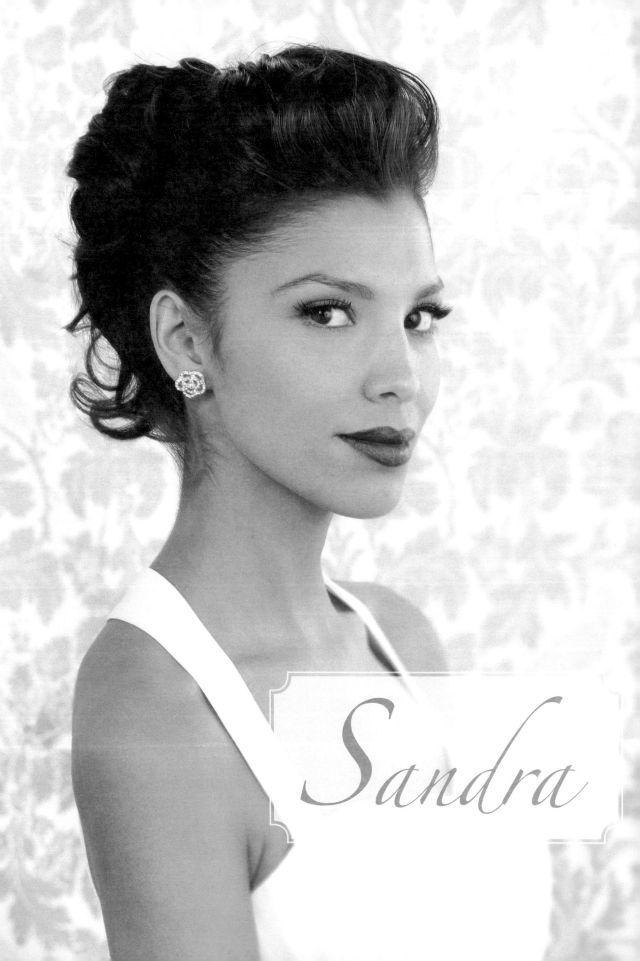

Sandra

The **Sandra** hairstyle design is great for the fun, 1950s style wedding. It also looks great with a tulle covered, A-line prom dress.

Its inspiration is the rockabilly pompadour, an indelible hairstyle of the past. The hairstyle itself is simple to execute and can be done quicker when you are rushed for time.

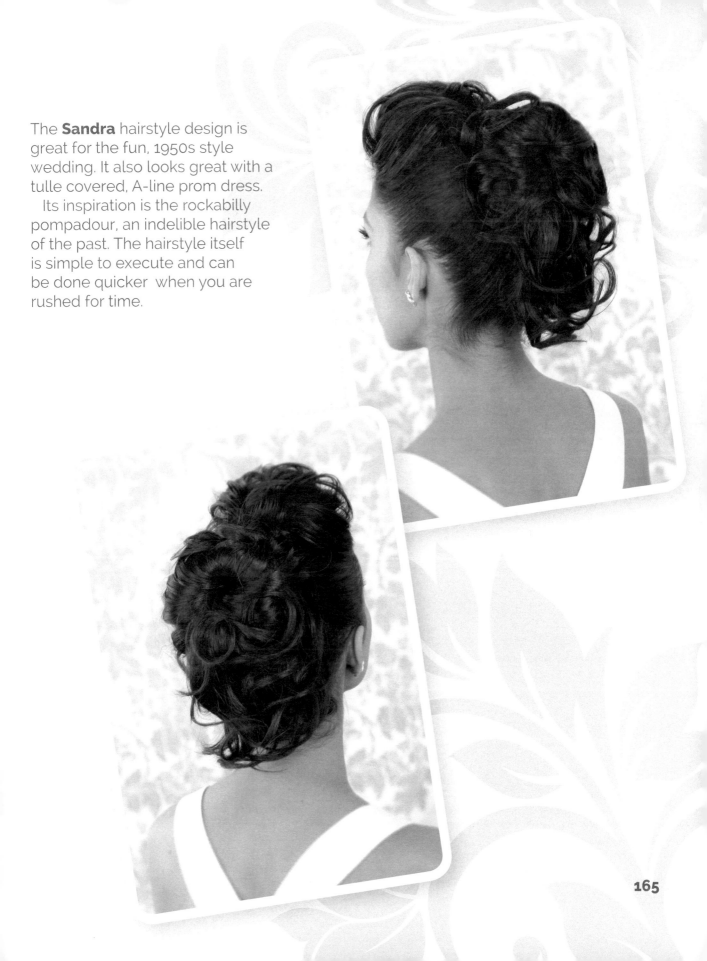

Supplies

volume spray
thermal hair setting spray
hairspray
pomade
hair dryer

hot rollers
carbon tail comb
round vent brush
grip bob pins

ripple hair pins
hair clips
large rubber bands
hair filler

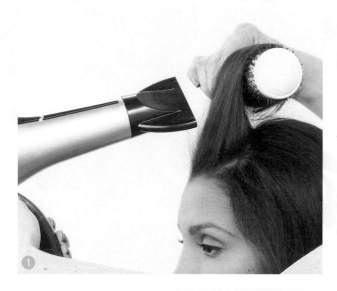

1 Prep using the steps described on page 22 for setting product into the hair. Use a volume blow-dry to eliminate any unruly growth patterns and add volume to the front hairline.

2 Set the entire head in medium hot rollers. Around the hairline just above the ears, roll the hot rollers up toward the crown.

3 Roll the hair at the back of the head in a basic bricklay pattern.

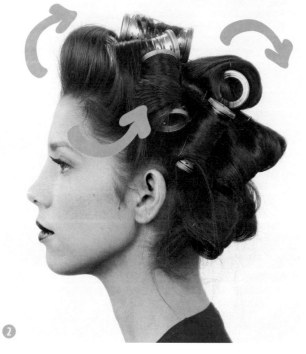

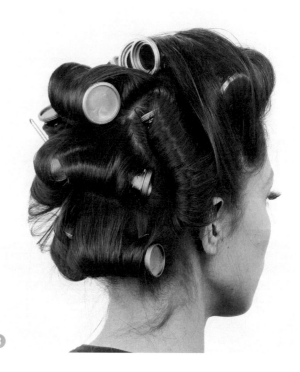

4 Remove the hot rollers after they have cooled. You will be working in 2 main sections for the Sandra. To separate the sections, use the tail comb to draw a triangle section. Start above the outer corner of the left eyebrow. Part in a diagonal back to a point that lines up with the nose and sits about 4-5 inches back from the hairline. Finish the third point of the triangle above the outer corner of the right eyebrow.

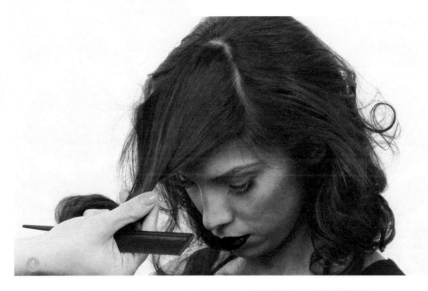

5 Using the directions on page 27, put the rest of the hair that makes up the back section into a high ponytail.

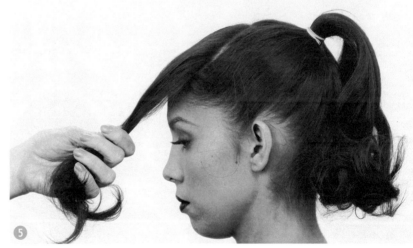

6 For this hairstyle you will want a small, oblong hair filler. See page 24 for a description of creating your own hair fillers. Holding the triangle section tightly forward over the forehead, grip pin the hair filler to the hair base. The back of it should line up with the back of the triangle shape.

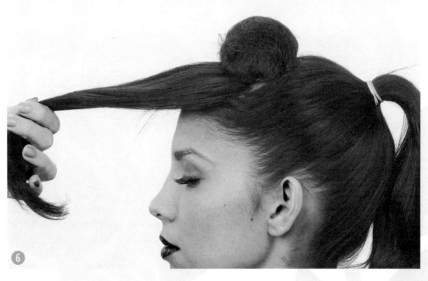

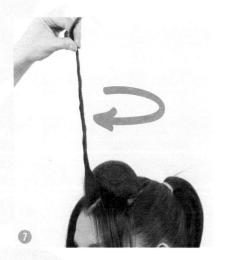
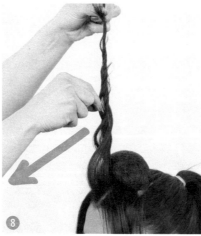
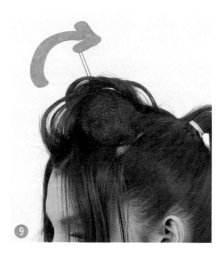

7 Working with the hair from the triangle section that is now hanging forward over the forehead, part out a ½ inch wide piece in the center. Draw the hair straight up and twist the piece several times.

8 Keep a tight grip on the ends with your left hand. With your right hand, beginning toward the ends, pinch small bunches of hair and pull them gently to loosen them away from the twist. Do not pull so hard that you pull them completely out. The hair should still be secure in the twist. Continue loosening small bunches along the twist so that the look is balanced.

9 Gently lay the hair section back over the hair filler. Use ripple pins to hold the section in place and keep it from unraveling temporarily. This will make it easier to change your arrangement if needed before the hairstyle is permanently secured in place.

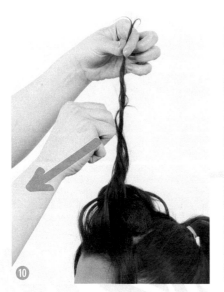
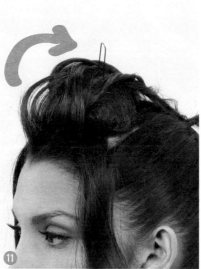
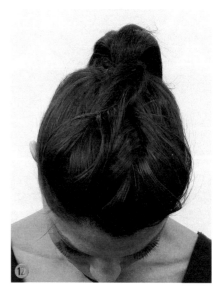

10 Continue to part out ½ inch wide pieces. Draw the hair straight up and twist. Pinch small bunches of hair and pull them gently to loosen them away from the twist.

11 Gently lay the hair section back. Use ripple pins to hold the section in place and keep it from unraveling.

12 Continue to follow steps 7-9 until you have used all of the hair in the triangle section to cover the hair filler. Once you have the front arranged the way you want it, place grip bob pins through into the hair filler below to secure the hair where needed and remove the ripple pins.

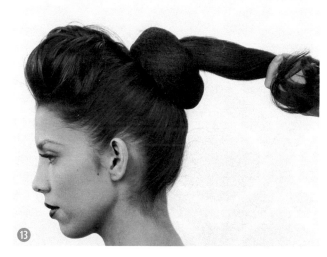

⑬

13 Pull the ponytail through a doughnut shaped hair filler and secure the hair filler to the base using grip bob pins. In this scenario, I used a hair padding from Sharon Blain Education that is perfect for this hairstyle. See the resource section in the back of the book. You can also create your own using the steps on page 24.

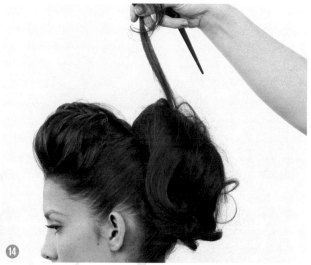

⑭

14 With a little pomade on your fingers, separate out bits of curl. Back-comb the curl to lock the hairs together. Smooth it with a comb and arrange the curl to cover the hair filler.

15 Use ripple pins to hold the curl in place temporarily. Continue step 14 on the rest of the hair, covering the hair filler completely. When you reach the lower half of the hair filler, let some of the ends hang loosely down below. Grip bob pin everything in place to secure the hairstyle.

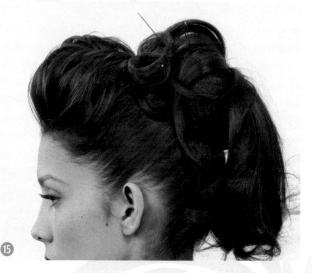

⑮

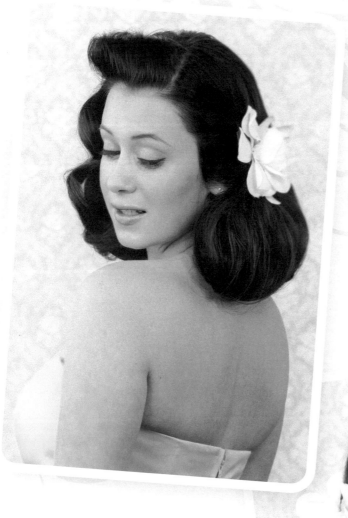

The inspiration for the **Lena** hairstyle comes from the silhouette of 1950s actress Diana Dors' hair. A cascade wave comes down the side near the face and the bottom perimeter is styled into a contained, low-hanging faux bob.

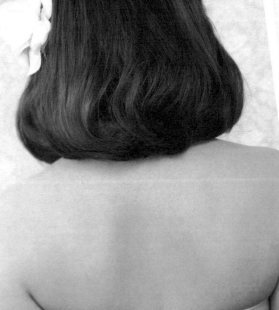

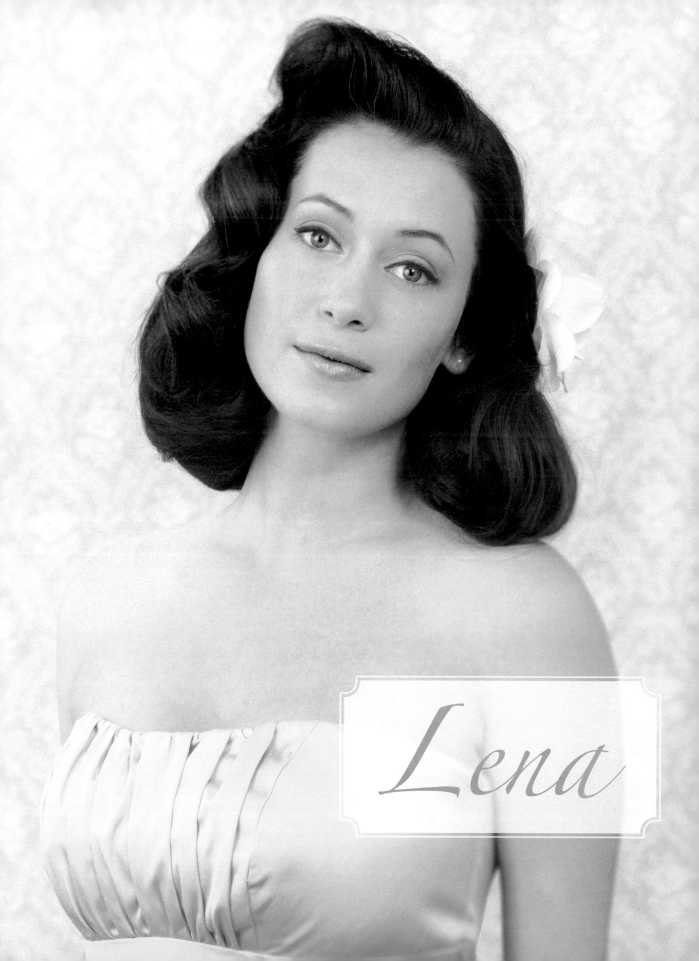

Lena

Supplies

volume spray	hot rollers	grip bob pins
thermal hair setting spray	carbon tail comb	ripple hair pins
hairspray	wide tooth comb	hair clips
pomade	natural bristle grooming brush	hair nets with elastic

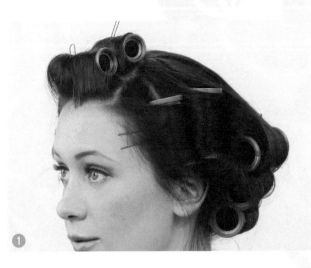

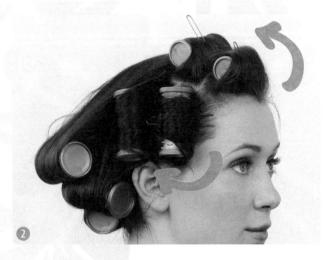

1 Prep using the steps described on page 22 for setting product into the hair. Use a volume blow-dry to eliminate any unruly growth patterns and add volume to the front hairline. Set a 3x3 inch section above the forehead in 2 small hot rollers parallel to the forehead rolling back.

2 Set the sides in medium hot rollers perpendicular to the floor rolling back away from the face. Set the rest of the hair toward the nape of the neck in large hot rollers.

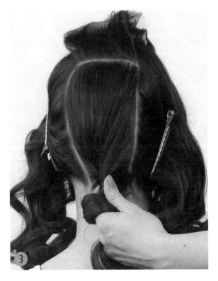

3 Leave the 2 small hot rollers at the top and remove the rest of the hot rollers after they have cooled. Separate the hair into the back section. Use the tail comb to draw a centered horseshoe shaped part that is 2-3 inches wide at the base of the neck, widens over the occipital bone, and ends at the back of the crown. Clip everything else out of the way. Note: There should be a 1 inch thick section surrounding the hot rollers to be used later.

4 Back-brush this entire portion of hair to lock the hairs together and spread the shape.

5 Smooth the hairs over the top with a brush.

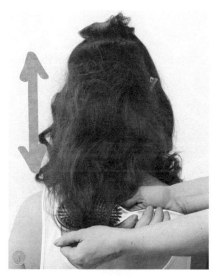

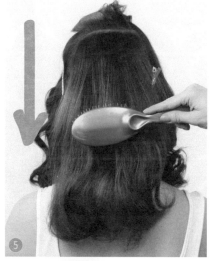

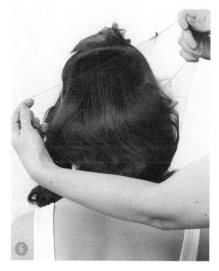

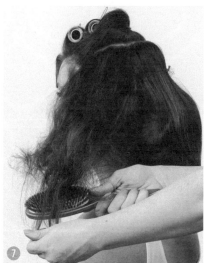

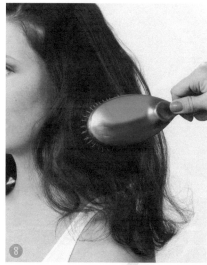

6 Use a bouffant sized hairnet with elastic in a color that matches the hair. Wrap the hairnet around the bottom of the hair mass to encase it. Grip pin the hairnet to the hair at the scalp to hold it in place.

7 Using all the free hair to the left, leaving the 1 inch section above it out, back-brush this entire portion of hair.

8 Smooth the hairs over the top.

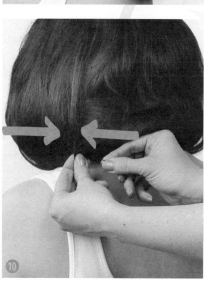

9 Wrap a hairnet around the bottom of the hair mass to encase it. Grip pin the hairnet to the hair at the scalp.

10 Use a grip pin to enclose the space between the 2 hair nets at the bottom.

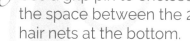

11 Repeat these steps on the right side. Using all the free hair to the right, leaving the 1 inch section above it out, back-brush the entire portion of hair. Smooth the hairs over the top. Wrap a hairnet around the bottom of the hair mass to encase it. Grip pin the hairnet to the hair at the scalp. Use a grip pin to enclose the space between the back hair net and the right at the bottom.

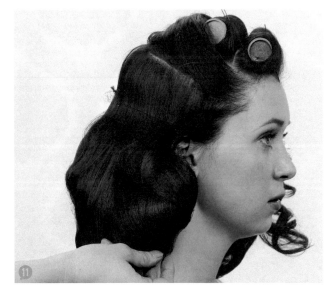

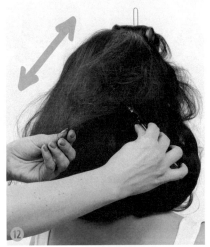

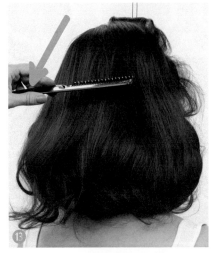

12 Next, unclip the 1 inch section that is between the lower pieces just worked with and the hot rollers on the top. Starting with the back, back-comb to lock the hairs together and spread the shape.

13 Arrange the hair to hide the hairnet underneath and smooth the hairs over the top.

14 Take loose ends that are hanging lower than the hairstyle, back-comb the ends to lock them together.

15 Turn the ends under to hide them and grip pin them in place to secure. Lightly spray the back with hairspray.

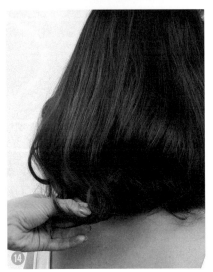

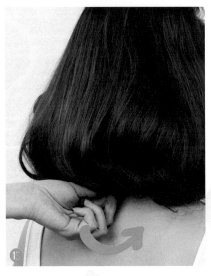

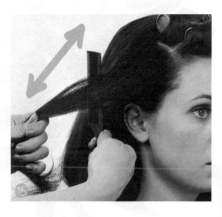
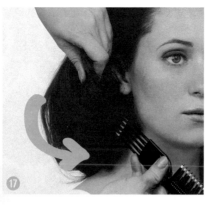
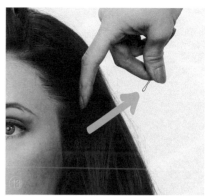

16. Move to the right side. Using the 1 inch thick section on the right side, back-comb to lock the hairs together and spread the shape.

17. Arrange the hair to hide the hairnet underneath. Round the hair over the front to create a sweep in toward the ear. Smooth the hairs over the top. Turn the ends under to hide them and grip pin them in place to secure.

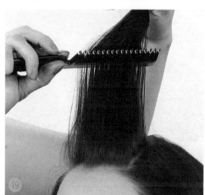

18. Repeat steps 16 and 17 on the left side. Then, using your finger, press the side so the hair lays tightly against the scalp and direct the hair back with pressure to accumulate behind the ear. Grip pin it in place to secure.

19. Remove the last 2 hot rollers at the top. Comb the curls in one mass straight up from the scalp. Back-comb the section to start spreading the wave and locking the hairs together.

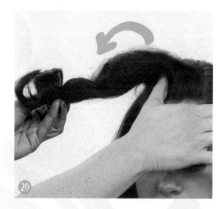

20. Place your thumb at the base and bring the section over to the right side of the head. The thumb placement helps define the arch in the hairline above the eyebrow.

21. Comb and arrange the wave down the side of the face. Grip pin it in place to secure the shape.

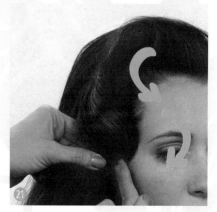

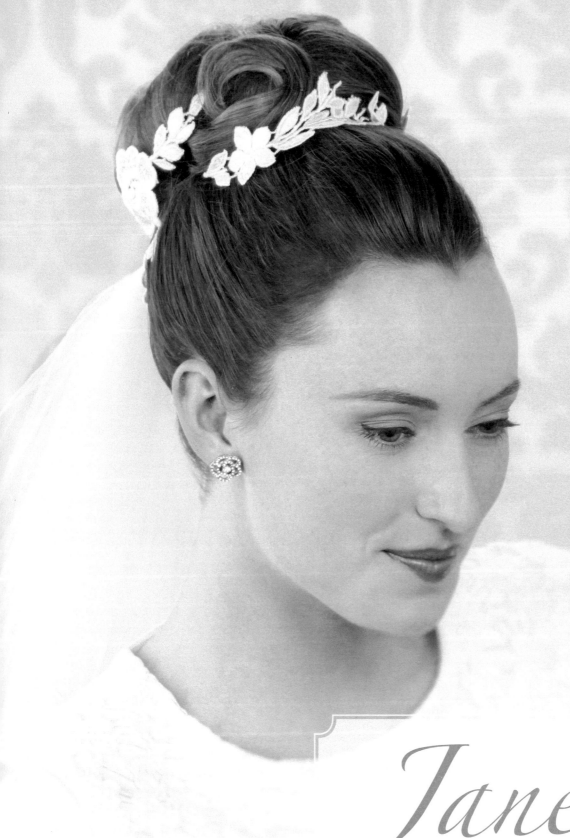

Janet

The **Janet** hairstyle, like the Judy hairstyle ahead in the book, is inspired by a 1960s bridal hair design booklet that featured many large, ornate elements.

The design is impactful, but simple to execute. It looks great by itself or decorated around the base with lace or flowers.

The hair filler inside the style also makes it possible to style any size you would prefer.

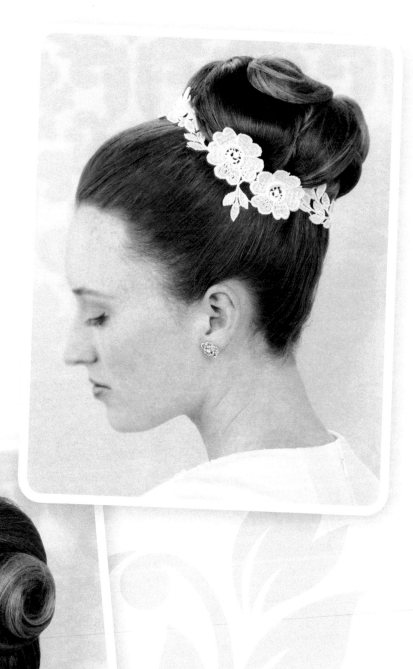

Supplies

thermal hair setting spray
hairspray
pomade
hair dryer
1" curling iron

carbon tail comb
wide tooth comb
grip bob pins
ripple hair pins
duckbill clips

hair clips
large rubber bands
hair nets with elastic
hair filler

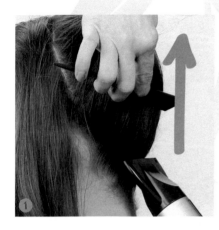

1 Vigorously massage the hair at the scalp while you blow-dry to eliminate any strange growth patterns especially at the front hairline. Base direction blow-dry at the nape of the neck and around the hairline by the ears to avoid droops at the hairline. See page 23 for more on base direction blow-drying.

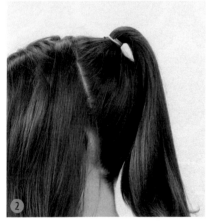

2 Using the steps described on page 27, gather the hair at the back half of the head into a high ponytail that sits at the back of the crown. Tip: Stand in front of the client with their head down while gathering the hair. This puts your fingers wrapped around the back of the ponytail which will allow for better grip and control.

3 Bring back the rest of the hair to the base of the ponytail.

4 Using the steps on page 27, attach the first ponytail and this new hair together into 1 large ponytail. Using this double ponytail technique will make for a stronger all day hold, especially on thick hair.

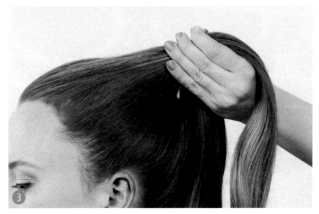

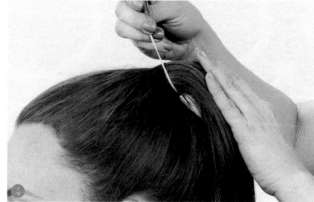

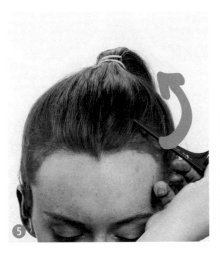
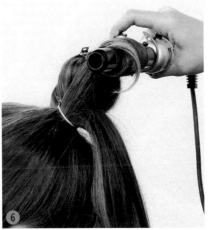
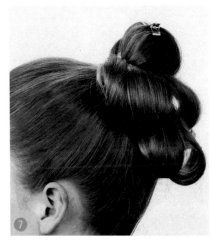

5 Smooth the outside or crust of the hairstyle. Insert the tail comb gently under the outer hairs that are on the exterior and move the comb back and forth using the tail to press and massage the hairs to align with each other.

6 Use the 1" curling iron to curl the ponytail in small sections.

7 Clip the curls to cool.

8 When cooled, separate the ponytail into 2 equal section with a part down the middle and clip to the sides.

9 Place a dense, doughnut shaped hair filler over the base of the ponytail. In this scenario, I used a hair padding from Sharon Blain Education that is perfect for this hairstyle. See the resource section in the back of the book. You can also create your own using the steps on page 24. Insert grip pins at the base all the way around the hair filler to secure it to the scalp.

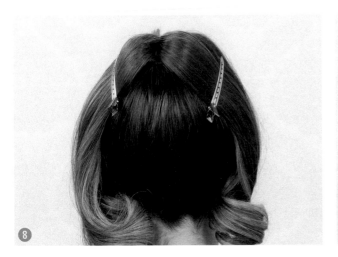
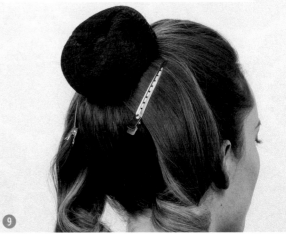

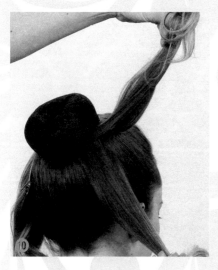 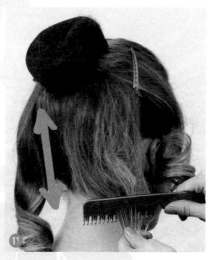 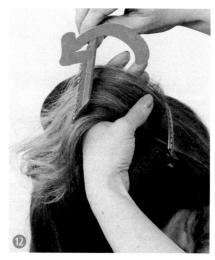

10 Unclip the right half of the ponytail and separate it into 2 equal pieces.

11 Back-comb deeply into one section to start spreading the wave and locking the hairs together. Extra back-combing is recommended to bring out the fullness.

12 Smooth the outer side for appearance.

13 Use a smaller bun sized hairnet with elastic and wrap the hairnet around the hair mass to encase it.

14 Gather any superfluous hairnet at the base and grip pin it to hide it under the hair filler.

15 Now rotate and manipulate the piece to cover the lower part of the hair filler. Play with the angle and configuration. Insert grip pins through the piece and into the hair filler below to secure it.

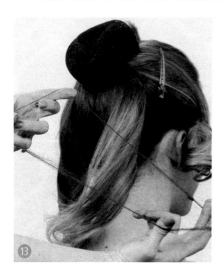 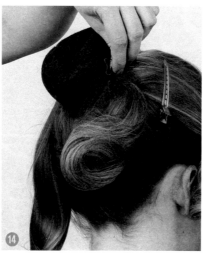 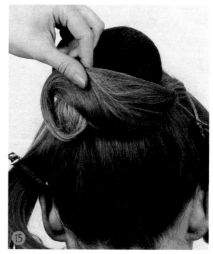

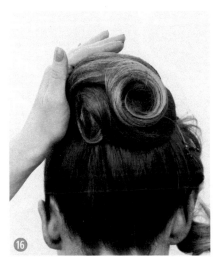
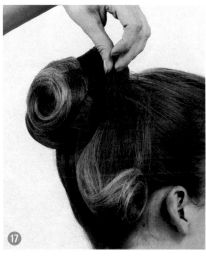
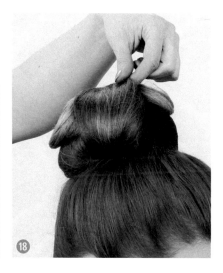

16 Unclip the left half of the ponytail and separate it into 2 equal pieces. Repeat steps 11-15 with one piece on the left and arrange it to sit just above the already finished piece at the bottom of the bun.

17 Go back to the right side and style the other half of the right side using steps 11-15.

18 Arrange this right piece to sit above the last piece that was styled. You are creating a stacked effect that will go up the bun as you cover it.

19 With the final piece from the left side, use steps 11-15 to cover the last portion of the hair filler.

20 Arrange the ends in a pin curl shape. Be sure that the entire hair filler is now covered. Grip pin everything into the hair filler underneath.

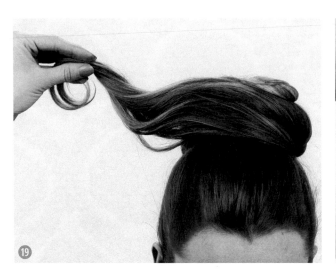
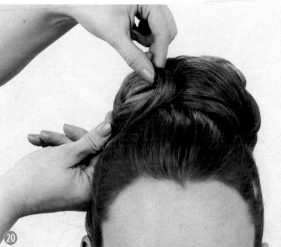

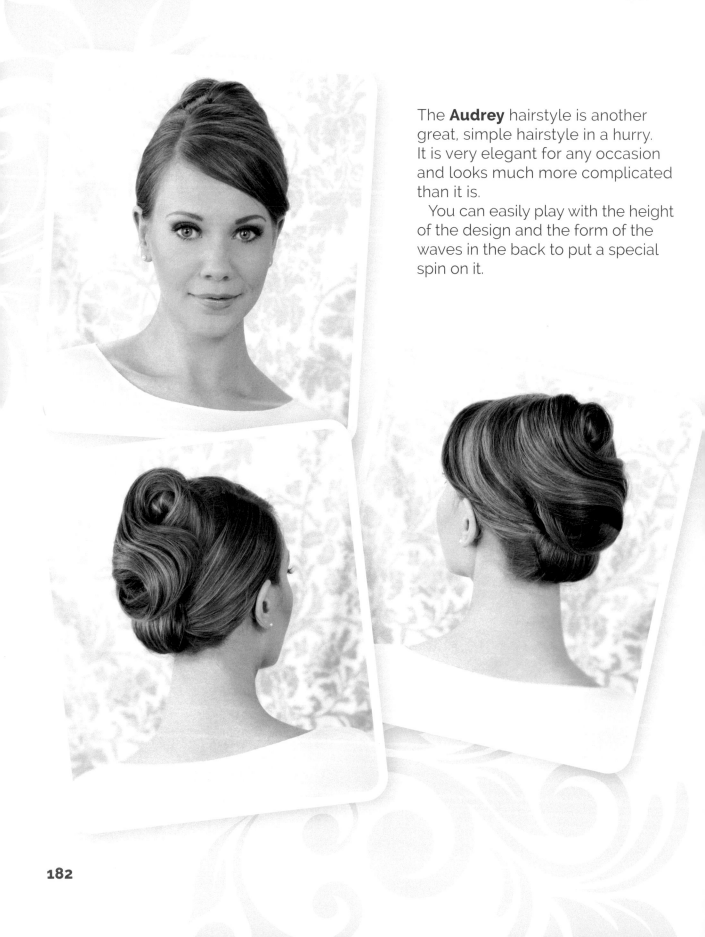

The **Audrey** hairstyle is another great, simple hairstyle in a hurry. It is very elegant for any occasion and looks much more complicated than it is.

You can easily play with the height of the design and the form of the waves in the back to put a special spin on it.

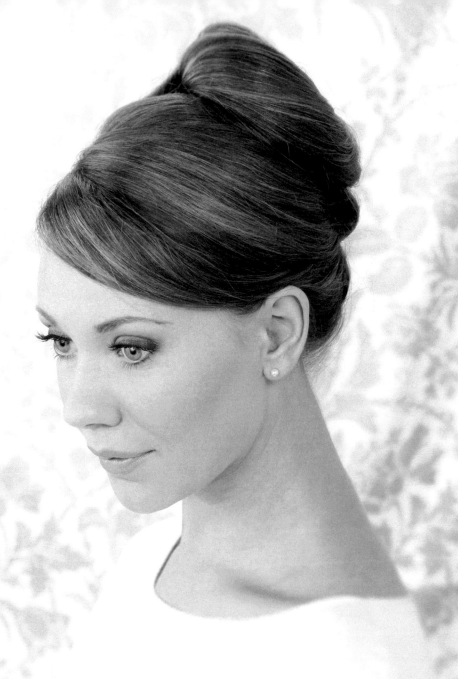

Audrey

Supplies

thermal hair setting spray
hairspray
pomade
1 ½" curling iron
carbon tail comb

wide tooth comb
natural bristle grooming brush
loop and tail styling tool
grip bob pins

ripple hair pins
duckbill clips
hair clips
small rubber bands

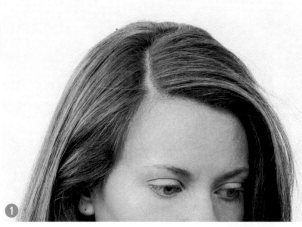

1 Prep the hair using the steps described on page 22 for setting product into the hair and adding volume to the hairstyle. Use the steps described on page 23 to set the part over so that it lies above the outer corner of the right eyebrow.

2 Part out a circular section at the back of the crown that is about 4-5 inches in diameter. Put in a ponytail using a small rubber band.

3 Collect the rest of the hair leaving a small section of fringe out to be used later. If the part was placed properly above the right eyebrow and the first section was circular, when you collect the rest of the hair into a ponytail below the occipital bone, the partings from the first ponytail should now be covered. Secure the lower ponytail with a small rubber band.

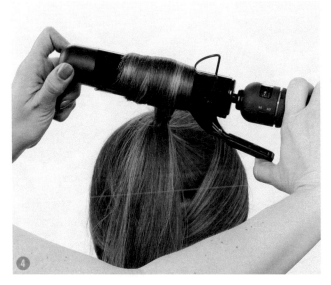

4 Curl the hair in the ponytail with a 1 ½" curling iron.

5 Clip the curls to cool.

6 Using the loop and tail tool, insert the tail down the center of the lower ponytail base between the scalp and the rubber band. Center the ponytail inside the loop. Pull the tail down and all the way through along with the ponytail to create a topsytail twist.

7 Using the same tool, insert the tail up from below through the center of the upper ponytail base. Center the ponytail inside the loop. Pull the tail up and all the way through along with the ponytail to create a topsytail twist.

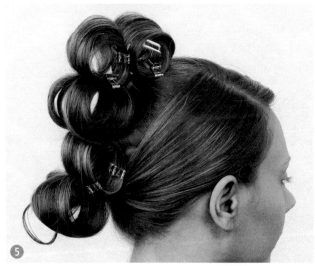

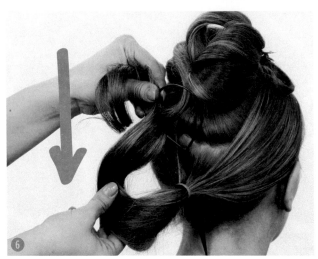

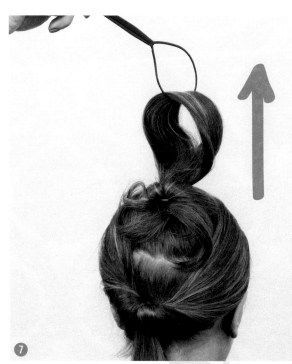

8 Back-brush deeply into the lower ponytail to start spreading the wave, add fullness, and lock the hairs together.

9 Smooth the visible side. Do not brush out the section, just smooth the outside. You need the tangles inside to help hold the form.

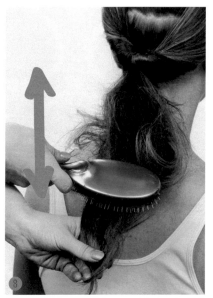
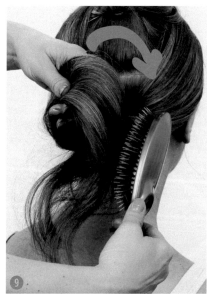

10 Flip the lower ponytail up and hold it up. Use grip pins to secure the lower portion of the ponytail into its base on either side.

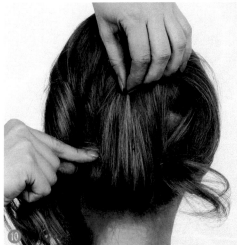

11 Now rotate, twist, and manipulate the piece up the right side of the head. Play with the wave and configuration to get the desired shape. Grip pin through the outer hair to the scalp hair underneath to secure it.

12 Repeat the steps on the upper ponytail. Hold the ponytail straight up and back-brush deeply into the ponytail to start spreading the wave, add fullness, and lock the hairs together. Smooth the visible side.

13 Flip the hair down and direct it to the left.

14 Rotate, twist, and manipulate the piece down over the back of the head. Play with the wave and configuration to get the desired shape. Grip pin through the outer hair to the scalp hair underneath to secure it.

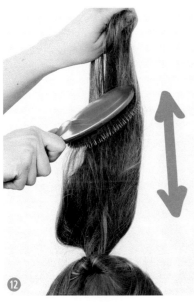

15 Move to the front and the small piece of the fringe section left out. Back-comb the fringe underneath to lock the hairs together. As you do this direct the hair to the left side a little at a time. This will help hold the side sweeping motion of the style.

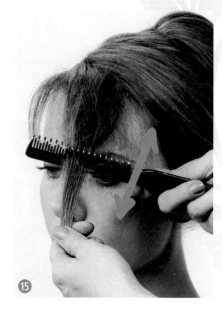

16 Smooth the visible hairs on top.

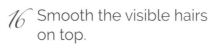

17 Holding the ends in your hand off to the side, give your hand a quarter turn down. This will spin the strands slightly under adding motion and form to the front. Grip pin the ends down behind the ear hiding the pins up underneath the outer layer of the hairstyle.

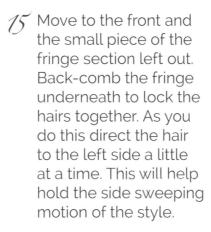

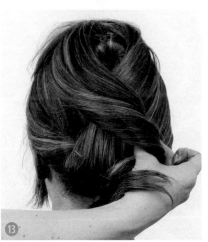

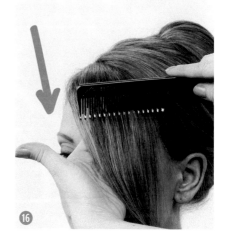

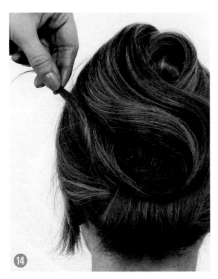

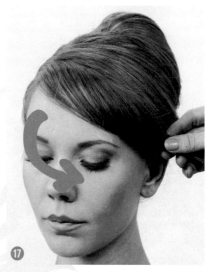

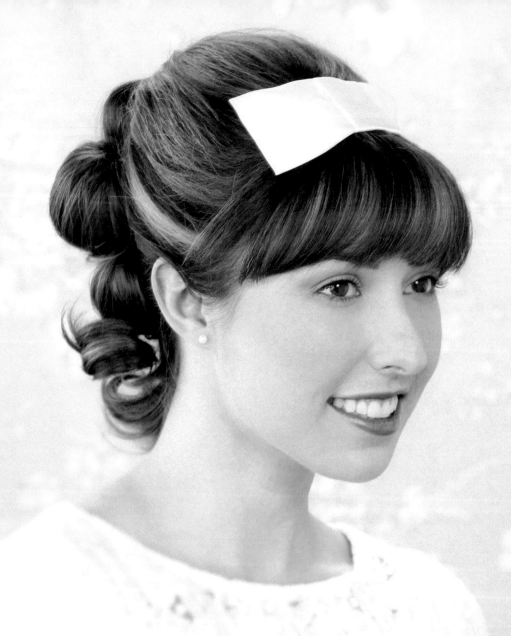

Judy

The voluminous bouffant came full circle by 1962. The **Judy** hairstyle draws its inspiration from a 1960s bridal hair design booklet that featured many large, ornate elements.

This design provides a simple, bouffant silhouette from the front and gorgeous detail from behind. If you are working with hair that is longer than this model's hair length, try tucking the ends into dry pin curls. It will still look lovely and capture the same feel.

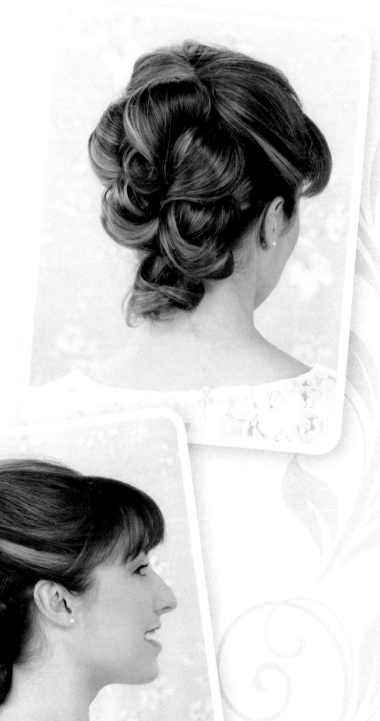

Supplies

volume spray	1" curling iron	ripple hair pins
thermal hair setting spray	carbon tail comb	duckbill clips
hairspray	wide tooth comb	hair clips
pomade	round vent brush	small rubber bands
hair dryer	grip bob pins	hair fillers

1 Prep using the steps described on page 22 for setting product into the hair. The hairstyle begins with all the hair at the back of the head and behind the ears.

2 This area is going to be separated into smaller sections strategically shaped so that each one covers the parting marks of the section before it. Start with an oblong section centered at the top. Secure it in a small rubber band.

3 The next piece is to the left. Include a small sliver of hair from above section 1, to the left of section 1, and below section 1. Secure it in a small rubber band. Notice that by including hair surrounding section 1, its partings are now covered.

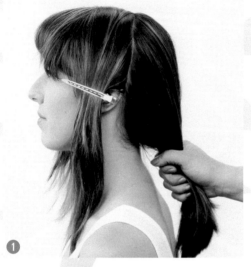

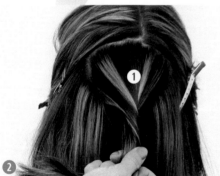

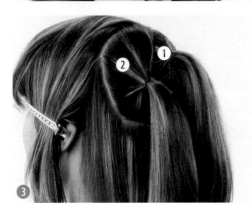

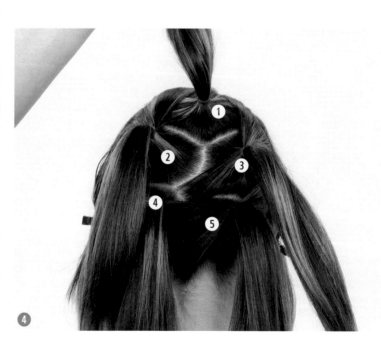

4 Section 3 is to the right of section 1 and slightly lower than section 2. It includes a small sliver above section 1, the right of section 1, and below. Secure in a small rubber band.

For section 4 on the left, note in image 3 that there is a small sliver of hair to the left of section 2. Include this small sliver, a sliver below section 2, and a small section below the left side section 3. The base shape will look like a long diamond shape. Secure with a rubber band.

Section 5 includes a small sliver of hair to the right of section 3, the hair left below section 3, and to the left and below section 4. Note in image 4, the bottom is now clean with no visible partings. Experiment a few times to get the configuration.

5 You now have 3 small ponytails in the back. Curl each one with the 1" curling iron.

6 Clip curls to cool.

7 To help with volume, place a long, thin hair filler over the top of this back section. See page 24 for more information on making your own.

8 At the front of the style back-comb thin sections running parallel to the forehead to lock the hairs together and add volume.

9 Lay each section back over the hair filler as you work. Use ripple pins to hold your work in place. Finish back combing so that the entire front and side section of hair are lying back and across the filler.

10 Smooth the outside.

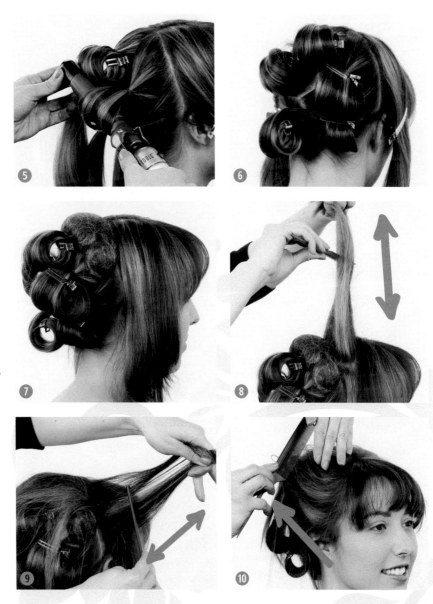

191

11 Use ripple pins to help balance the shape and hold the bouffant while you work.

12 Collect the ends gently in a group, twist, and secure at the scalp on the base of the first ponytail from step 2 to be hidden later.

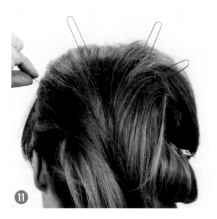
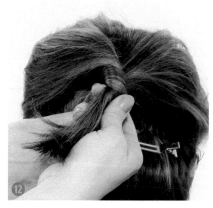

13 Move on to the back. For this hairstyle you will need 5 small, oblong hair fillers. See page 24 for a description of creating your own hair fillers.

Begin with ponytail 5 at the nape of the neck. Clip all the other ponytails out of the way. Hold ponytail 5 at a diagonal up away from the neck. Back-comb it to lock the hairs together and smooth the outer appearing side. Place a small, round hair filler over the base of the ponytail and secure it tightly with grip bob pins.

14 Bring the ponytail down over the hair filler. Use a ripple pin to spread the hair gently to cover the hair filler completely. Grip pin the hair around the base to secure it.

15 Work your way up the back and repeat steps 13 and 14 with each ponytail. A little out of order, ponytail 3 is the next one secured in it forms.

16 Note that the ends of the pieces are not hidden in the hairstyle. This model's hair length allows for a clean look without hiding the ends. If the client's hair is too long for this to look nice, arrange the ends in pin curls and secure.

17 Repeat the steps on ponytail 4 and ponytail 2 after that working your way backward.

18 Note that with the placement of the hair fillers and the ponytails covering the hair fillers, all of the partings in the back are being covered.

19 Throughout the style, use ripple pins to temporarily hold hair sections while you arrange the hairstyle. For added security, hair sewing as described on page 26 will ensure that the hair stays in its place throughout the day.

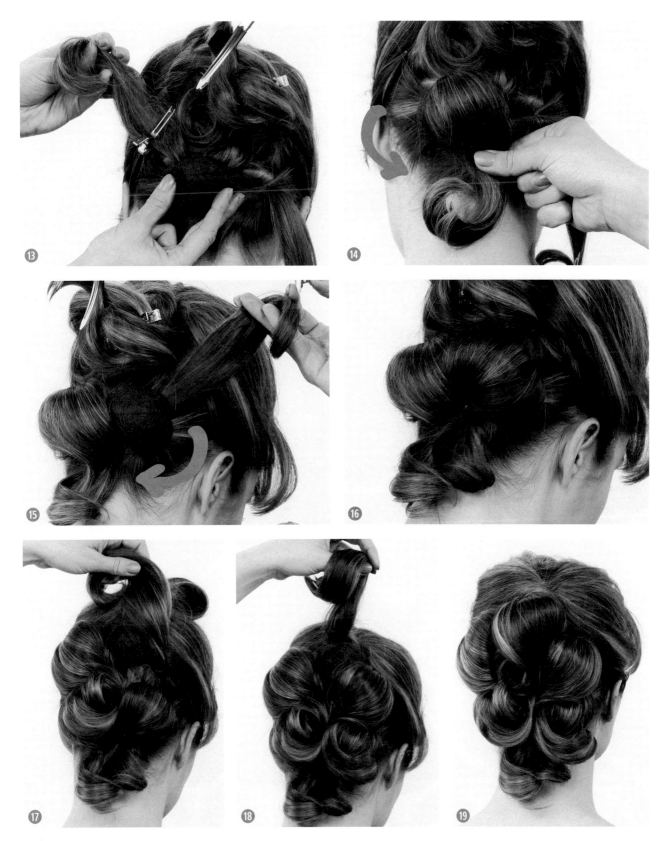

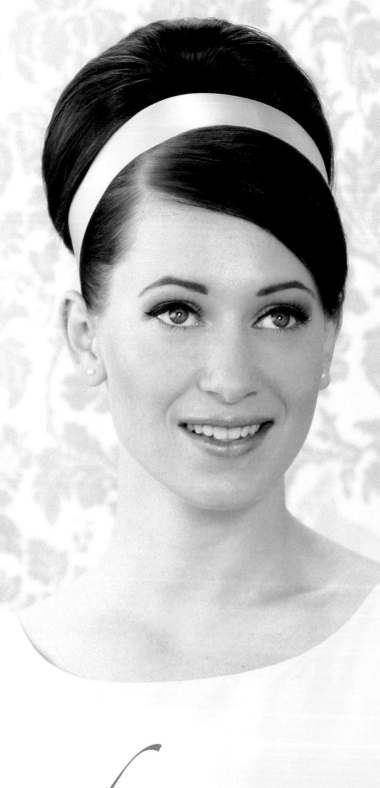

Linda

The **Linda** hairstyle and the Susan on the pages after are two different takes on the same silhouette. They are designed for the girl who wants Breakfast at Tiffany's hair.

The Linda is a more sleek, contemporary version. Its simple design makes it also a faster hairstyle to execute when you are rushed for time. It makes a great bridesmaid hairstyle for a 1960s wedding, when the bride is getting a more ornate look like the Susan.

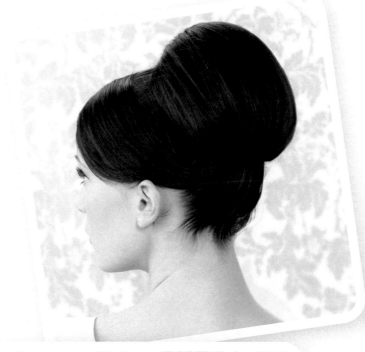

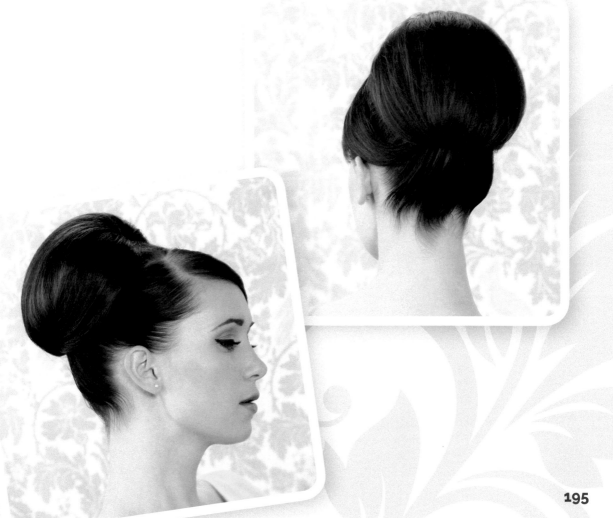

Supplies

thermal hair setting spray
hairspray
pomade
hair dryer
1 ¼" curling iron

carbon tail comb
wide tooth comb
natural bristle grooming brush
crochet loop tool
grip bob pins

ripple hair pins
duckbill clips
hair clips
small and large rubber bands

1 Prep using the steps described on page 22 for setting product into the hair. Use the steps described on page 23 to set the part so that it lies above the outer corner of the right eyebrow.

2 Curl all the hair loosely with the 1 ¼" curling iron.

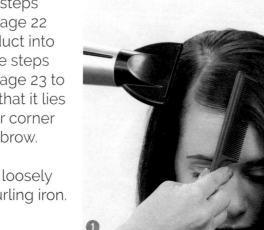

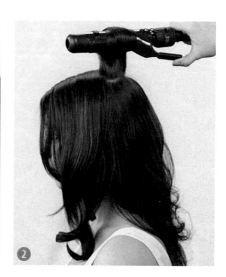

3 There are 3 main sections to the Linda hairstyle. At the front, separate out a 1x2 inch piece to the right of the part. To the left of the part, separate a 2 inch deep section stretching over to above the left eyebrow. Everything else in this hairstyle will go in a ponytail.

4 Using the steps described on page 27, gather the hair at the back half of the head into a high ponytail that sits at the back of the crown. Tip: Stand in front of the client with their head down while gathering the hair. This puts your fingers wrapped around the back of the ponytail which will allow for better grip and control.

5 Steps 5-11 below describe the method for creating the spray effect at the front of the bun of this hairstyle.

Attach a grip pin to a large rubber band. Attach the pin horizontally to the hair at the scalp about an inch forward from the base of the ponytail.

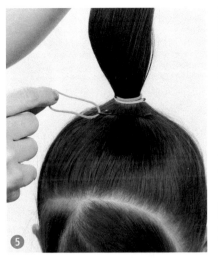
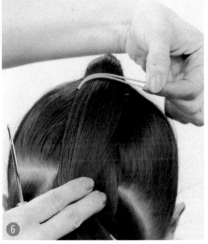
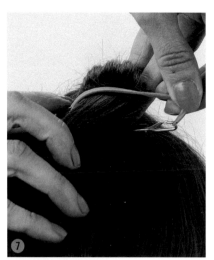
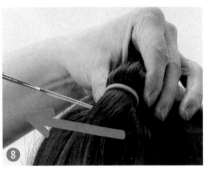
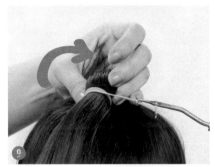
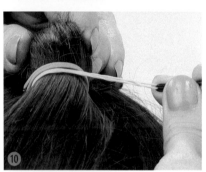

6   Take the entire ponytail and bring it over the top of the head to lay on top of the grip pin. Wrap the rubber band over the top of the ponytail.

7   Weave the latch hook through the hair at the scalp and in front of the grip pin and grab hold of the rubber band.

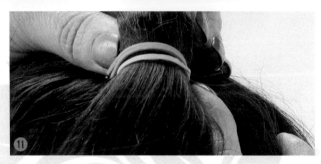

8   Pull the rubber band back through the hair at the scalp.

9   Wrap the rubber band one more time over the ponytail.

10   Attach a grip pin to the rubber band.

11   Secure the rubber band end under the ponytail close to the first grip pin.

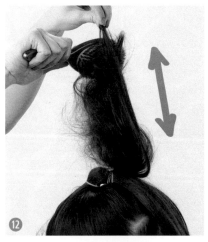

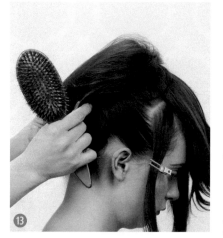

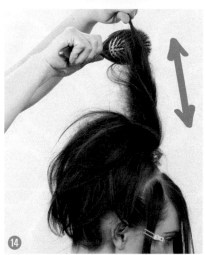

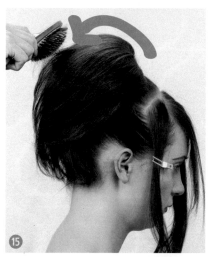

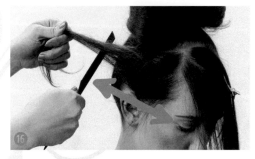

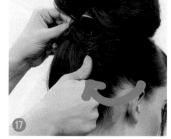

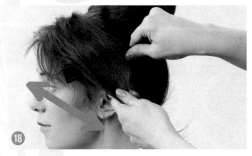

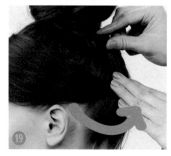

12 Working in 3 or 4 sections, separate a piece out of the ponytail. Back-brush it to lock the hair together and add volume.

13 Bring it back behind the head over the base of the ponytail.

14 Continue to separate out pieces of the ponytail and back-brush for volume.

15 Lay all of these sections back over themselves and smooth the outer hairs with a brush for appearance.

16 Gently clip this hair mass up out of the way for the next steps. Move to the front. Back-comb the piece to the right of the part to lock the hairs together. As you do this, direct the hair to the right a little at a time. This will help hold the side sweeping motion of the style. Smooth the hairs on top for appearance.

17 Bring the ends around the back, below the ponytail base and grip pin it in place.

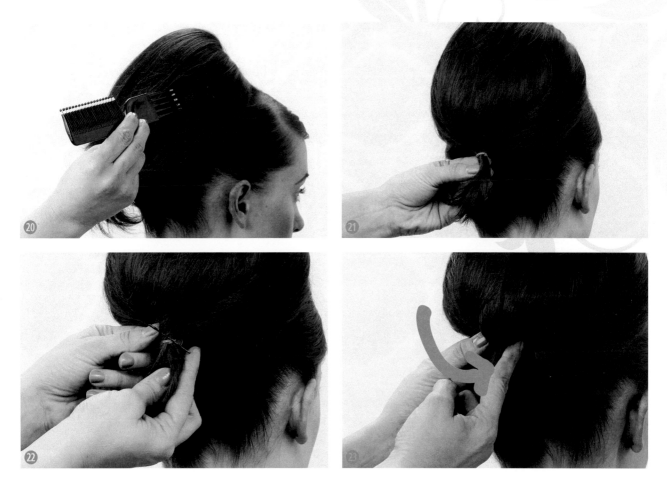

18 Repeat these steps with the section of hair to the left of the front part. Back-comb the piece to lock the hairs together. As you do this, direct the hair to the left a little at a time. Smooth the hairs on top for appearance.

19 Bring the ends around the back, below the ponytail base and grip pin it in place.

20 Working with the hair mass from steps 12-15, place it back to cover over the ponytail base and the pins. Use a pick or wide tooth comb to manipulate the mass into a symmetrical, rounded shape.

21 Pinch the ends of hair together to hold the round mass and secure the ends with a small rubber band.

22 Insert a grip bob pin through the rubber band.

23 Turn the rubber band and ends under to be hidden under the hair mass. Insert the grip bob pin to the hair at the scalp underneath to secure in place. Use grip pins as needed throughout the edges of the hair mass to secure the hairstyle.

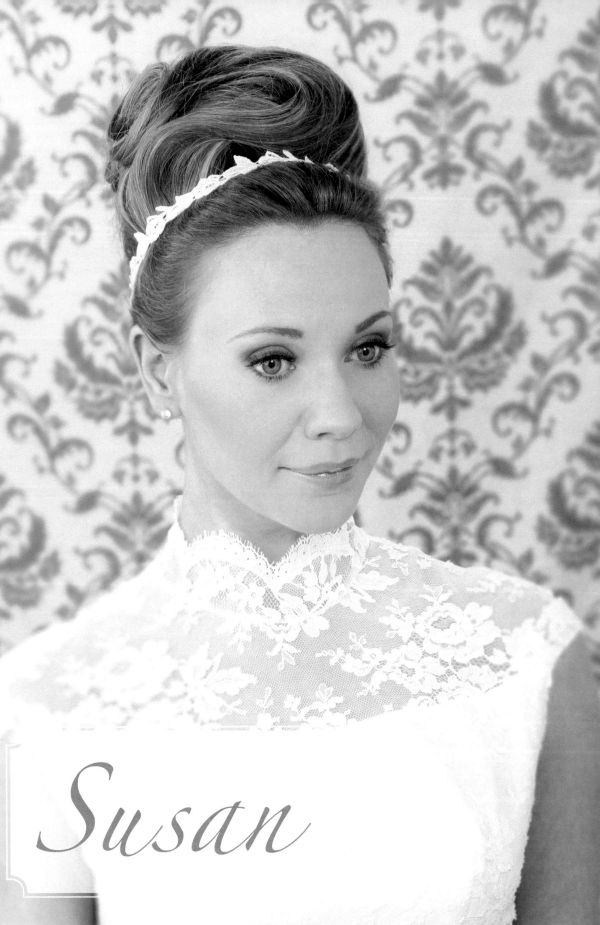

Susan

The **Susan** hairstyle, like the Linda before it, is designed for the girl who wants a Breakfast at Tiffany's silhouette.

The base of the hairstyle provides a good start to a 1960s high bouffant and the shape and detail can be customized in different ways to suit the hair length and texture.

Balance and proper pinning is important to the longevity of the hairstyle. Make sure the base underneath is well anchored to ensure the entire hairstyle holds up.

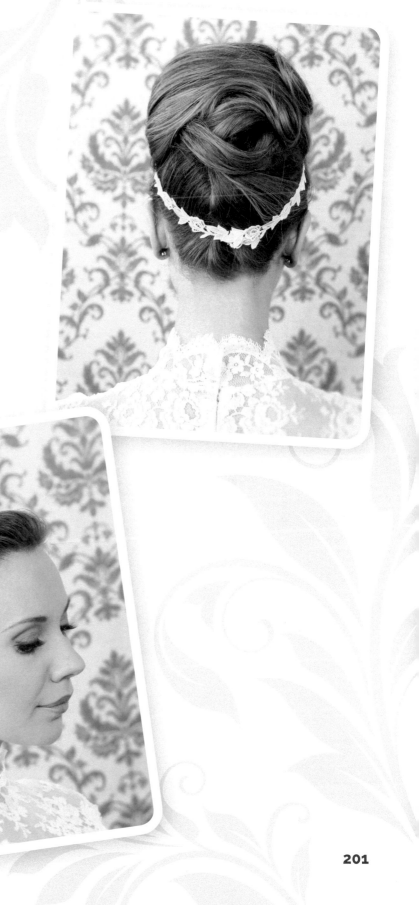

Supplies

volume spray
thermal hair setting spray
hairspray
pomade
hair dryer
hot rollers

carbon tail comb
styling brush
wide tooth comb
round vent brush
natural bristle grooming brush
grip bob pins

ripple hair pins
duckbill clips
hair clips
small rubber band
thin beading cord elastic

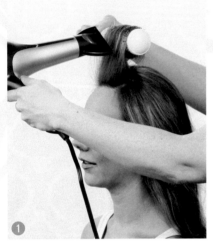

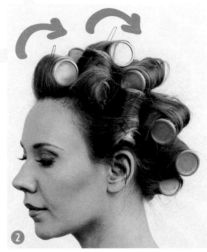

1 Prep using the steps described on page 22 for setting product into the hair. Use a volume blow-dry to eliminate any unruly growth patterns and add volume to the front hairline.

2 Set the entire head in medium hot rollers. Roll the hair in a basic brick-lay pattern.

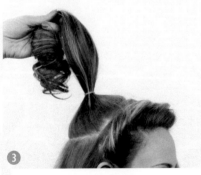

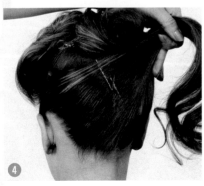

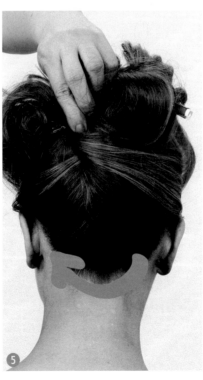

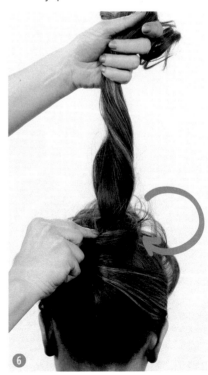

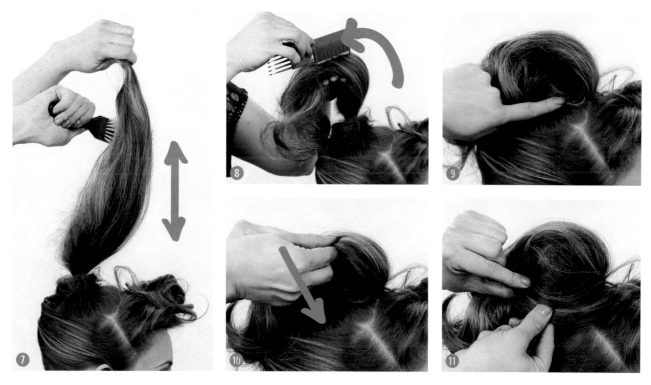

3 After the hot rollers have cooled, remove all of them. Separate a circular section at the back of the crown with a 4 inch diameter and secure the ponytail with a small rubber band. Clip it out of the way.

4 Collect the hair below the circular section and to the left and right of it. Brush it tightly directing it to the right. Insert grip bob pins to secure the center.

5 Create a French twist with this hair at the back.

6 Wrap the ends of the hair from the French twist around the base of the ponytail from the circular section in step 3. Grip pin them in place to secure.

7 Back-brush the ponytail to lock the hair together and add volume.

8 Smooth the outer hairs for appearance.

9 Fold the ponytail forward and then back over the base of the ponytail. Insert grip bob pins to secure it in front of the ponytail base.

10 Use your fingers on either side of the mass, spread the sides gently over and down to the scalp.

11 Grip pin to secure.

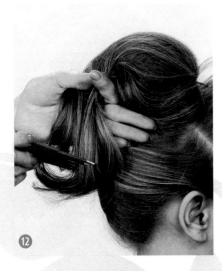

12 Gently holding the ends of the ponytail so as not to disturb the hair mass you just created.

13 Comb and arrange the ends into a wave shape and cover the back of the hairstyle. Grip pin to secure.

14 Brush the last of the hair above the forehead up into one section.

15 Bring it back over the hair mass and use ripple pins to temporarily hold it in place.

16 Cut off a 2 foot long piece of thin beading cord elastic.

17 Using the elastic as a head band, wrap it over the top of the head and tie into a knot at the nape of the neck.

18 Use grip bob pins to secure it in place and keep it from slipping.

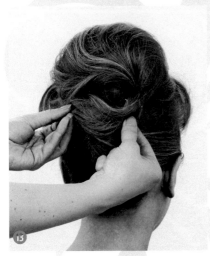

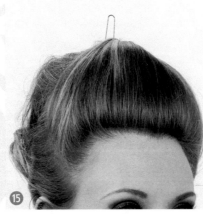

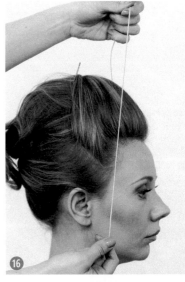

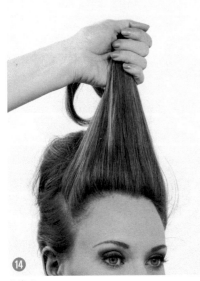

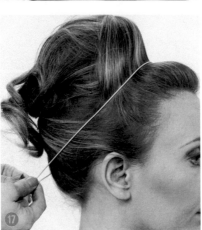

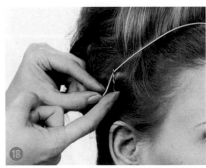

19 Remove the ripple pin freeing the top hair section. Manipulate the hair to the left and then around to the right to create a waving swirl.

20 Use a ripple pin to help form and manipulate the wave shape.

21 Arrange the ends in pin curls and grip pin them in place to secure. Strategically add grip pins throughout the style to secure it.

22 Wrap a thin piece of lace over the thin beading cord elastic to hide it and finish the look.

23 Grip pin the lace to secure it.

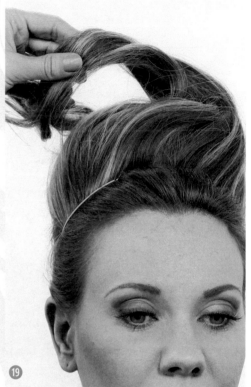

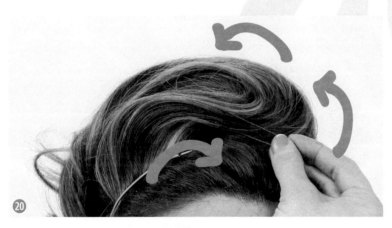

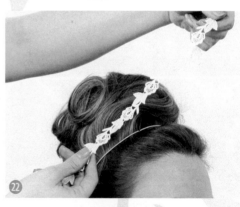

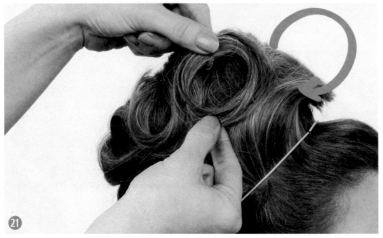

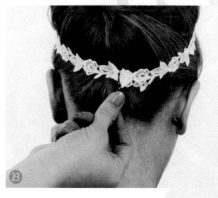

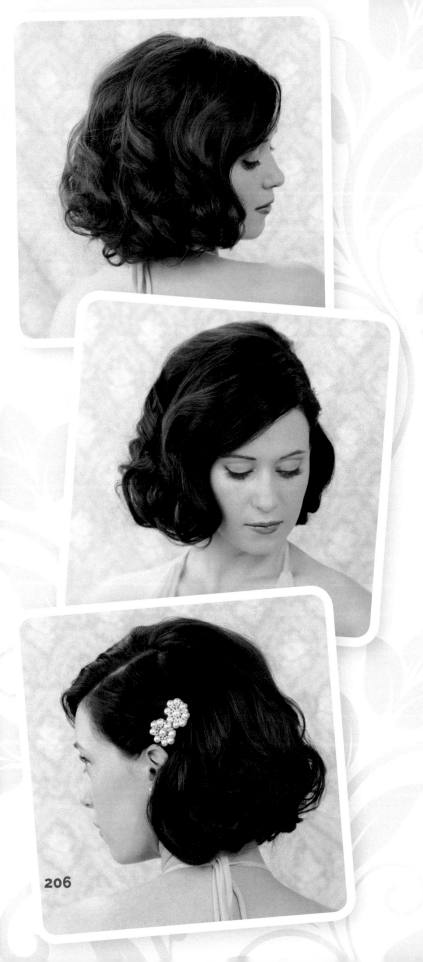

The design of the **Patricia** hairstyle is a modern, soft faux bob interpretation of the short bouffant popular in the early and mid-1960s. It is inspired by the sultry actresses that wore the hairstyle so well like Elizabeth Taylor and Sophia Loren.

The key to keeping this hairstyle soft and accessible for today's bride is the looseness of the curls. They should not be brushed together in a smooth clump, but rather left separate from each other. The curls at the front of the style also cascade a bit into the right of the face and close to the eye to keep the look contemporary and young.

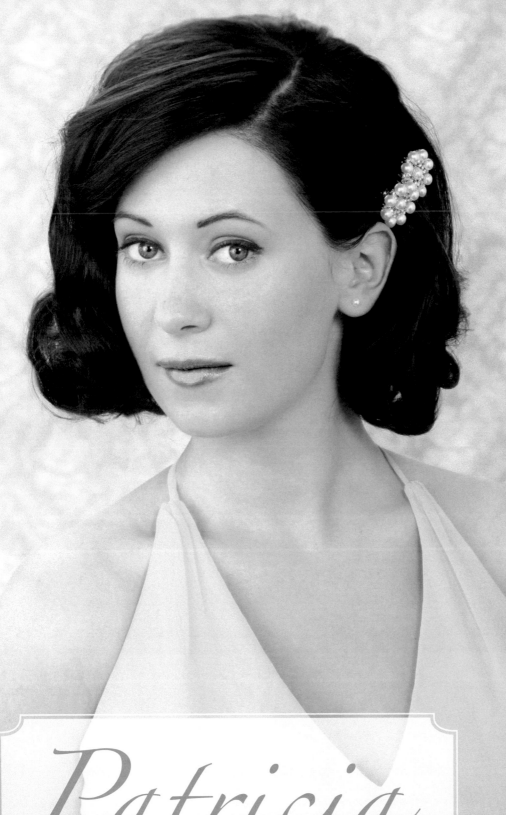

Patricia

Supplies

volume spray
thermal hair setting spray
hairspray
pomade
hair dryer

1" curling iron
1 ½" curling iron
carbon tail comb
round vent brush
styling brush

grip bob pins
ripple hair pins
duckbill clips
hair clips
hair net with elastic

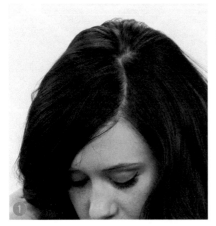
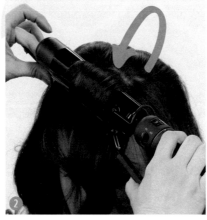
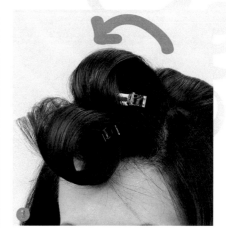

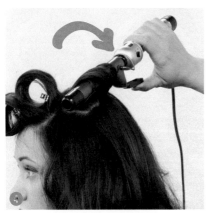

1 Prep using the steps described on page 22 for setting product into the hair. Use a volume blow-dry to eliminate any unruly growth patterns and add volume. Set the part over so that it lies above the peak of the left eyebrow.

2 With the 1 ½" curling iron, curl the fringe area at an angle forward toward the forehead.

3 Clip the curls to cool.

4 With the 1" curling iron, curl the rest of the hair down the opposite direction.

5 Curl in a basic brick-lay pattern all the way around the head and clip the curls to cool.

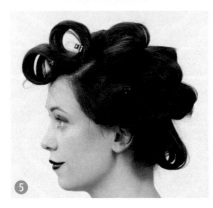

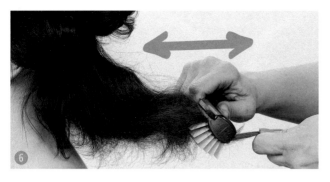
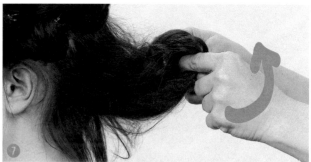

6 Next, you are going to create a hair filler using the existing hair. Remove the clips from only the lower set of curls. Separate a section out encompassing all of the hair at the base of the neck. Using the steps described on page 25, back-brush the hair to lock the hairs together and add volume.

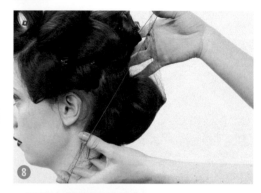

7 Roll the hair, ends first, up and over themselves toward the lower half of the occipital bone.

8 Wrap a hair net around the hair mass.

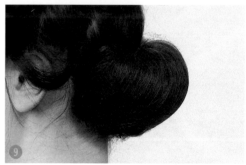

9 Fluff the mass as needed and grip pin the hairnet to the scalp.

10 Now remove the clips from the next row of curls on the back of the head. In thin sections running parallel to the shoulders, back-comb an inch at the base of the scalp to lock the hairs together and add volume. Lay the hair back over the hair filler created in steps 6-9.

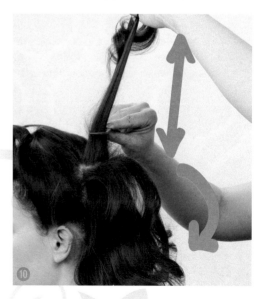

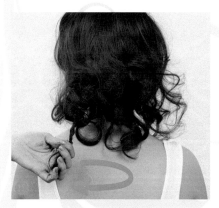
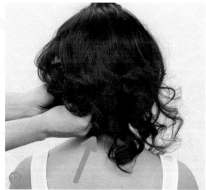
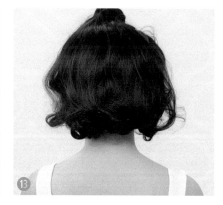

11 Using a small amount of pomade on your fingers, separate the curls and define them. On the first lower row, a piece at a time, twist the ends together and insert a grip bob pin to the end of the curls.

12 Pin the ends up underneath into the hair mass to start forming the faux bob.

13 Work across the back of the hairstyle until there are no more free ends.

14 Remove the clips from the next layer of curls. At the left side of the hairstyle, above the ear, use your finger to press the hair against the scalp to hold it in position. Use a grip bob pin to secure the side.

15 Manipulate the curl hanging down from this left side to curve in toward the ear. Then twist the ends together and insert a grip bob pin to the end of the curls.

16 Pin the ends up underneath into the hair mass. Work your way around to the right side of the hairstyle, pinning the ends under for the faux bob. Repeat step 14 to pin back the right side the same way as the left.

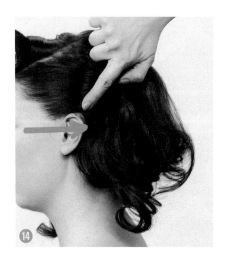
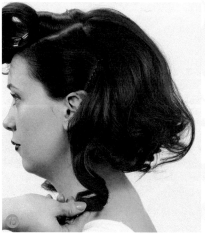
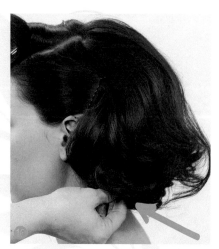

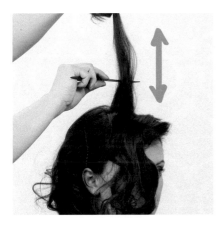

17 Remove the clips from the large, forward curls at the top. In thin sections running parallel to the forehead, back-comb an inch or so at the base of the scalp to lock the hairs together and add volume.

18 Spread the hair and lay it over the back, right side of the hairstyle maintaining the body of curl.

19 Continue to separate out thin sections of hair and back-comb for volume while maintaining the curl.

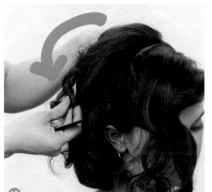

20 Manipulate, arrange, and lay them over the right side of the style. Grip pin the sections to secure.

21 When you have reached the last section to the right of the part, back-comb directing the hair over to the right as you go.

22 Smooth the hair on top for appearance.

23 Direct and manipulate the hair around the face to curve in toward the cheek. Secure with grip bob pins.

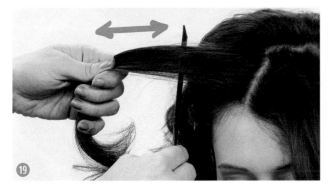

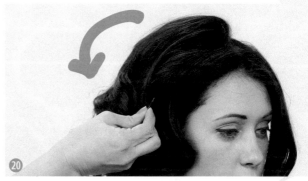

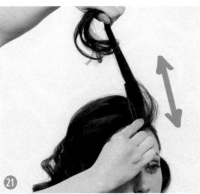

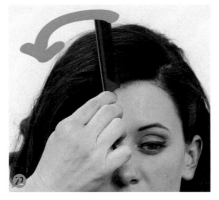

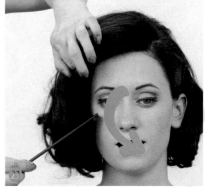

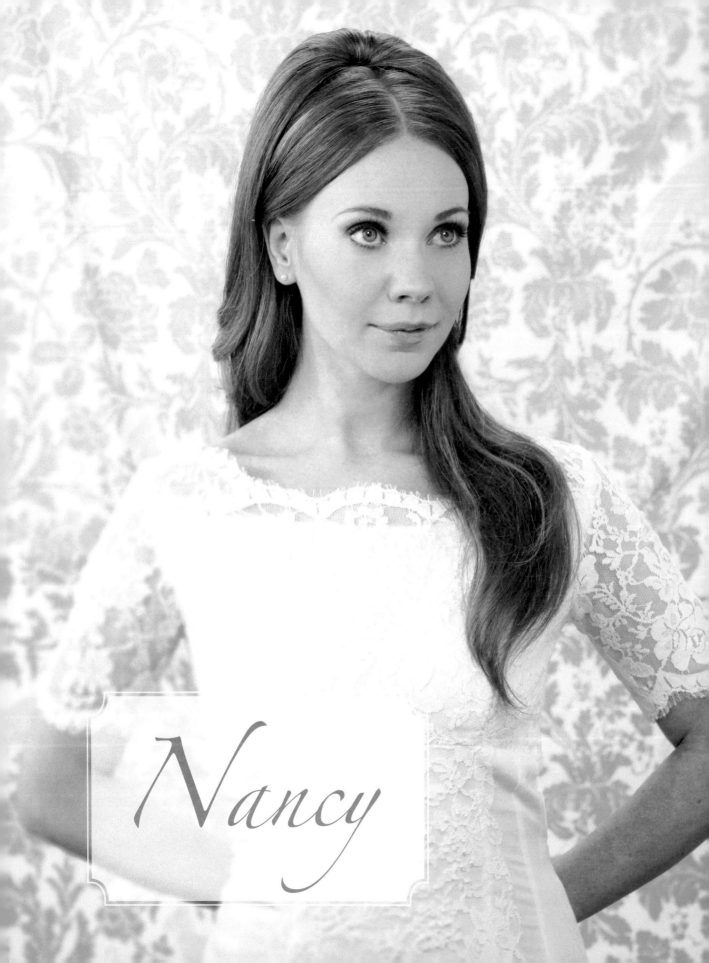

Nancy

The **Nancy** hairstyle is both one of my favorites in this book and one of the simplest to execute. It is inspired by the changes in women's hair fashion around 1965. Girls were growing their hair out longer and I have come across a number of wedding images from the late 60s in which the brides wore simple, chic down-dos such as this.

For a 1960s wedding, this style is both impactful and delicate. The height is not overdone, but there is no mistaking its roots in the history of style.

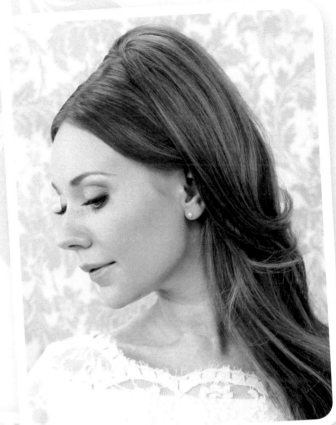

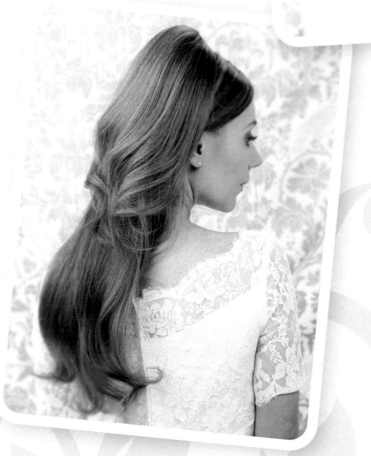

Supplies

thermal hair setting spray
hairspray
pomade
hair dryer
hot rollers

carbon tail comb
wide tooth comb
round vent brush
styling brush
loop and tail styling tool

grip bob pins
ripple hair pins
duckbill clips
small rubber band

1 Use the steps described on page 17 to prep the part. Spray the base of the hair at the scalp with thermal setting spray.

2 Use a base direction blow-dry to set the part so that it lies directly down the middle.

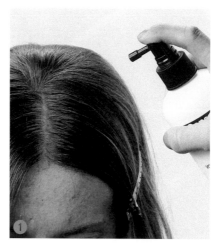

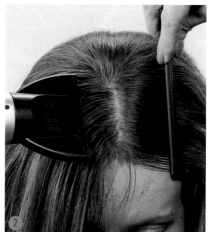

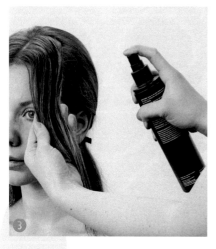

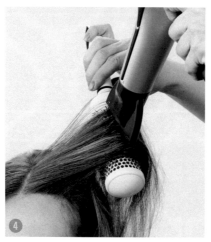

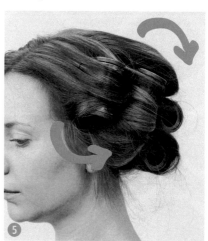

3 Prep using the steps described on page 22 for setting product into the hair.

4 Direct the hair back away from the face as you blow-dry prep.

5 Set the hair low in large hot rollers rolling back away from the face.

6 Part out a circular section that stretches from behind the right eye around the back of the crown and to behind the left eye and is about 4-5 inches tall. Put in a ponytail using a small rubber band.

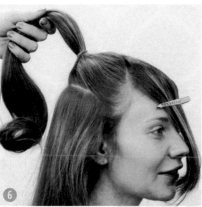

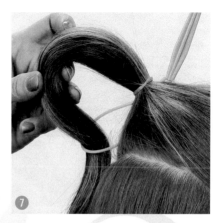

7 Using the loop and tail tool, insert the tail up from below through the center of the ponytail base. Center the ponytail inside the loop.

8 Pull the tail up and all the way through along with the ponytail to create a topsytail twist.

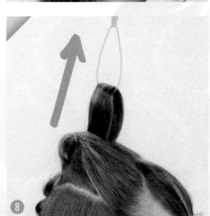

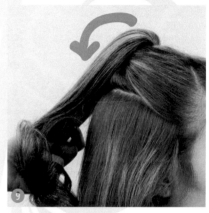

9 Bring the ponytail back and clip it for later use.

10 With a 1 inch wide section of hair behind the ear, create a small scalp or French braid that follows down at the hairline for about 2 inches.

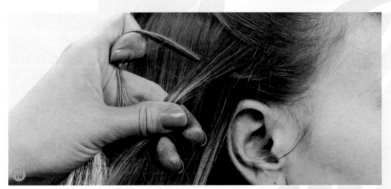

11 Use a small grip bob pin or 2 to secure the braid to the hair at the scalp.

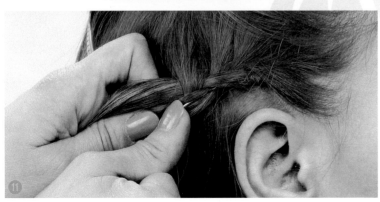

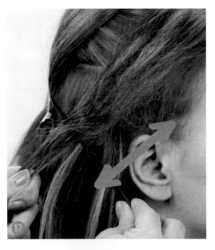

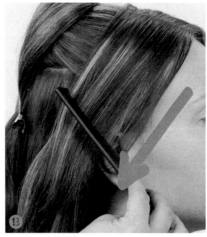

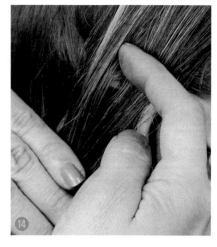

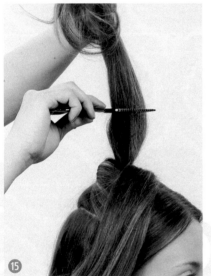

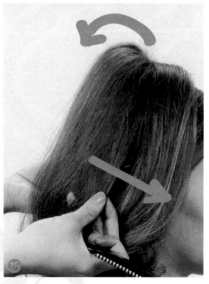

12 Move to the front. Back-comb the piece to the right of the part to lock the hairs together. As you do this, direct the hair to the right a little at a time. This will help hold the side sweeping motion of the style.

13 Smooth the hairs on top for appearance.

14 Secure the hair to side by pinning it flatly with the small grip pin penetrating through to the small braid behind the ear.

15 Working in 3 or 4 sections, separate a piece out of the topsy tailed ponytail. Back-comb this section to lock the hair together and add volume.

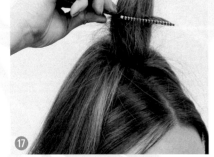

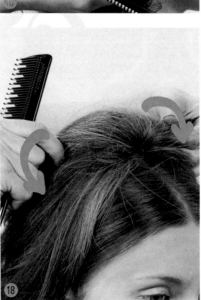

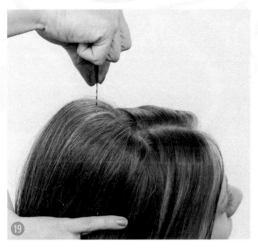

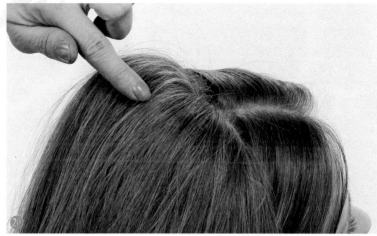

16 Bring it back behind the head over the base of the ponytail.

17 Continue to separate out pieces of the ponytail and back-comb for volume.

18 Lay all of these sections back over themselves and smooth the outer hairs with a brush for appearance.

19 Use small grip bob pins to secure this section.

20 Press the grip pin down in, but not so far that it flattens the volume.

21 See the description on page 29 for hiding grip pins. Use the ripple pin to guide the hair over the grip bob pin.

22 Use the ripple pin to refine and manipulate the hair smoothly.

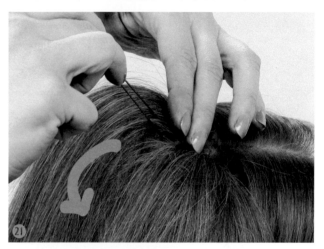

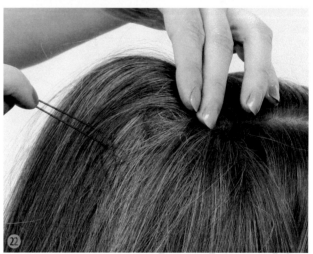

Anatomy

Apex - the highest point of the head

Crown - top of the head, area that would be surrounded if wearing a crown

Occipital Bone - situated at the back and lower part of the skull, curves down toward neck

Fringe area - refers to the area above the forehead where bangs are normally situated

Nape - the back of the neck, lowest point of the hairline

Resources

Here is a short list of websites where you can find the tools found in this book.

For brushes, combs, grip pins, curling irons, tapered wands, small rubber bands and many more hairstyling supplies-
www.sallybeauty.com

Hair sewing supplies and premade hair fillers
www.sharonblain.com

Latchhook tool and beading elastic
www.joann.com

Topsy tails and hot sticks
www.amazon.com

Number 16 large rubber bands for ponytails
www.officemax.com

Image Credits

Every effort was made to find and obtain reproduction permission for images. If you feel an image has been printed here unlawfully, please contact HRST Books LLC and every effort will be made to rectify it. All images copyright Lauren Rennells and HRST Books unless credited below. P.2: family photo; p.3: Jennings Photography St. Louis; p.4, 13 antique store finds; p.8, 12, 13: istockphoto.com; p.8, 12 Studio Voutre Beauty, *Specialty Coiffures*; p.11 Norcross greeting cards; p.15 *The Queen Ladies' Newspaper and Court Chronicle* April 2, 1864.

Before

If you would like to reference the hair length each hairstyle was created with, here are images of the models before they were styled.

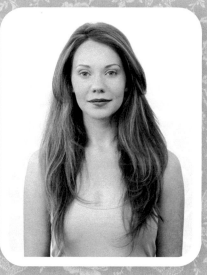
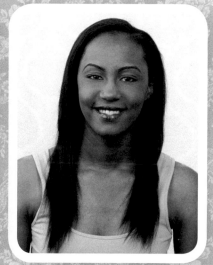
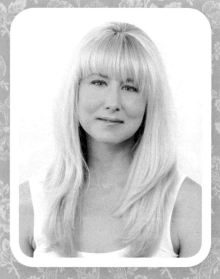
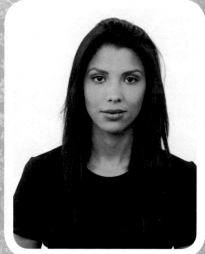
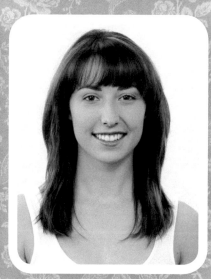
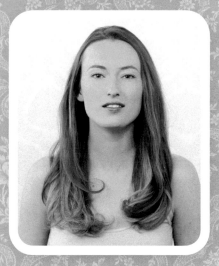
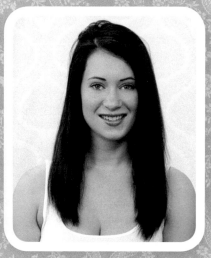
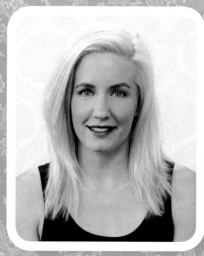

Discover more vintage beauty items…
at VintageHairstyling.com

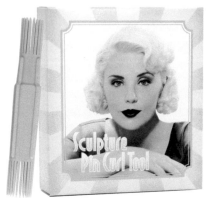

Sculpture Pin Curl Tool
MSRP $29.95 US

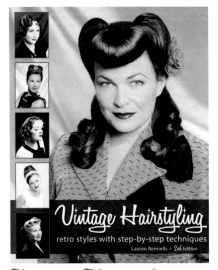

Vintage Hairstyling:
Retro Styles with
Step-by-Step Techniques
MSRP $36.95 US

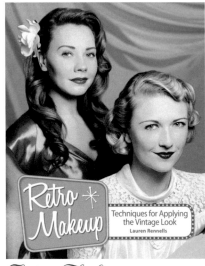

Retro Makeup:
Techniques for Applying
the Vintage Look
MSRP $23.95 US

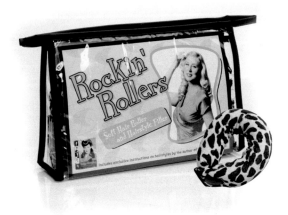

Rockin' Rollers
MSRP $22.95 US

Go to **www.vintagehairstyling.com**

❧ See our selection of retro hair tools, makeup, and educational material!

❧ Sign up for our email list to get notifications of special sales and exclusive tutorials!

❧ Find out when demonstration and classes will be available in your area!